# BIPOLAR LIFE

JASON TAFF

# BIPOLAR LIFE

## A JOURNEY FILLED WITH GOD

Tate Publishing & *Enterprises*

Published by Tate Publishing & Enterprises, LLC
127 E. Trade Center Terrace | Mustang, Oklahoma 73064 USA
1.888.361.9473 | www.tatepublishing.com

Tate Publishing is committed to excellence in the publishing industry. The company reflects the philosophy established by the founders, based on Psalm 68:11,
*"The Lord gave the word and great was the company of those who published it."*


*Cover design by Tyler Evans*
*Interior design by Lindsay B. Behrens*

Published in the United States of America

ISBN: 978-1-61663-031-7
Self-Help / Mood Disorders
10.03.15

# TABLE OF CONTENTS

# DEDICATION

This goes out to all of you who have been curled up in bed, fearing the day because it is too painful, to all of you who live with havoc in your minds while you try to work and live, to all the people who have compassion and need to learn about bipolar disorder and all that encompasses it. This goes out to you who seek a new beginning, for all who have felt pointless to the point that it was numbing and your nerves were on end, that even the vibrations of a clap you felt echoing through your skin causing irritability. While loud noises gave you a little fright, nowhere to turn, nothing to laugh at, despair growing on you like the frost on the trees on a winter night. To you whose cries were never heard. To you who have what feels like a sumo wrestler standing on your chest and a mountain high of people on your back while your goal is to climb up Mount Everest. To you who shout out and despair and look at your feet and cry for the shame you have carried way too long—the struggle is just way too deep, like rotting organs inside of you. The sun comes up. The sun goes down—over and over while you toil in the hot desert on your knees, begging for help. This book is for the people who can't figure out this phenomenon and want to help. This book is for any doctor anywhere who needs more insight. This book is for the Spirit of good, who is God, and for the One who allowed me to write this all for what I described above, because I originally wrote it for him, but he wanted it for you, so thank him: Jesus Christ!

# THANK YOUS

Thank you to all the books out there that educated me about bipolar disorder. Thank you, God, because... well, as my pastor would say, "You should thank God and then tell him what you're thanking him for." But, God, you know exactly what I'm thanking you for. Please, Lord. I don't want this to be a dramatic mess where I start to cry and get all emotional and thank you for how good you are and how you created me and how I could never be here if it wasn't for you. But I guess that's the way I feel. I guess this is where I should also be thanking my mom for how much she supported me throughout the years, through the hard times and the good times that we had to go through. And for my dad for being a solid rock in my life, and my brother and sister for simply existing with me and loving me in my life, and for all my friends for helping mold me to who I am today, and for my family pets keeping me full of joy when I hardly had any. And for my intermediate family, for all the special attributes they help give me in my life. For my uncle, Adam, and his wife, Sayuri, for being nice family members and for my uncle always pushing me toward education and teaching me how to study harder. "Thanks, man," I would say if I were actually thanking him. I would probably go on to say, "Thanks. I wouldn't have known about www.wikipedia.com and www.m-w.com and what all the different ideologies in life are if it wasn't for you." I thank him for the computer he once bought me and everything else I can possibly think of. That is if I were actually thanking him. And I thank my uncle, Dave, for helping my mom out when he did, or his sister, I should say, and for his kind generosity to allow all of us in his home, as often he does. I thank him for his kind spirit. I also go on to the other side of my family, my dad's side, and tell Grandma and Grandpa they're amazing and I want to visit them more often. I also tell the whole family I would like to see them all more often. But the thing is I don't want to get into a whole sloppy thank-you page, where I spill my guts out, but looks like I already did. Love you guys! Peace be with every single one of you. Oh, and this is where I should add in that person I forgot to thank. Uncle Dave, my dad's brother, and Uncle Don, my dad's other brother, and I guess if I was being all emotional I would say, "Dave, I love your jokes. Uncle Don and Aunt Fern, keep up the hard work." Then, of course, I would tell Krista and Ryan to hurry up and graduate and then come traveling with me or something extraordinarily fun. But this is not one of those gushy thank-you notes; this is simply something I'm making up to please people as if I am making a thank you note.-That's not the case at all I want to see you all soon, and take care until I do see you, and I'll probably even see you before you read this, but I grew up with all of you. I have been through life with all of you 'till this very day and plan on hopefully continuing that way. I have seen family, then I have seen us, and our family takes every nook and cranny, shoves it into one, and makes an explosive funhouse of excitement, triumph, times of sorrow, times of joy, hugs, laughter, yells and screams, great meals, relaxation, trips, amusement parks, camping, boating, work, crafts ... and, throughout it all, looked to every person who has ever been part of this family. Tell me you don't see love from every single one of them. If you do, that's a lie. I know there is—through the divorce, through the secrets, and through the pride—a secret prize inside. That prize is inside every one of us, and it connects us all. Stop screaming right now if you are, and remember we are family.

# INTRODUCTION

> Bipolar disorder affects approximately 5.7 million adult Americans or about 2.6% of the U.S. population age 18 and older every year.
>
> National Institute of Mental Health

> Bipolar is the sixth leading cause of disability in the world.[1]

A bipolar person laments about her mind racing so fast that she has to take notes to catch up with them. I thought, *Wow! I too have been making shorthand notes all summer, and my mind has been racing. I must be a little manic. But through it all, I still survive, and through it all I still feel better then I have the years before. I will recover, I will be healed, and I will survive!* This has been the mindset for me as I go through my recovery. Throughout this book, I will share stories with you and things I have learned, things I have done wrong while trying to overcome a mental illness I have called bipolar disorder. My hope is throughout this book there will be time to cry, laugh, get angry, and feel immense joy. My goal in writing this book is that we can all share in the glory I share in Jesus and that through our pain we will become stronger and better people. The goal of this book is also to inform and teach people what I know and have been through. I held nothing back as I wrote this book, and as it's read, I hope the readers will gain, if nothing else, that there is hope in all situations in life and we all can grow and help each other in community and know Jesus is God.

## FINDING MYSELF IN THE WAKE OF THE MOMENT

*A few months after I had received diagnosis that I was bipolar.*

At this time, I started getting into the Lord. I truly began to trust that he could and would heal me. So I gave my whole heart to him and believed he would heal me.

I hope that everyone will be healed and have a better life ahead of them. This will get you through it all: belief that there is a God and that he can and will heal.

I also thought the medication would heal me right away too. The doctor told me it could. So I took the medication and went to bed and prayed so hard that I would be healed the next morning.

The next morning I woke up. And one time I actually felt healed for a second. I shouted to the Lord and was so happy, and then I began to notice some of my symptoms again. I noticed my behavior, and it hadn't changed.

This happened a few more times, and then I began to realize, *Yes, Jason, this may take a while. The doctor said lithium sometimes takes a full year to have its full effect.* A year passed, and I had gotten better, but I still was suffering. This is why I believe God is healing me in time—because I'm still getting better. So maybe he used meds, plus time, plus his own love and grace to heal me, but, to me, meds and time are his grace. Thank you, God, for your grace! I will be healed completely. I earnestly, truly, full-heartedly believe that. He has a big plan for me, and he does for all people!

Satan would want me to stop believing when I didn't get healed right away from the meds. It was disappointing and very discouraging. I'll admit that. I'll also admit that God held onto me because I was at the end of my rope. I almost feel like I did let go, and I would have fallen even deeper if he hadn't caught me and lifted me up.

It would have been nice to be healed the day I started taking lithium. I think it was three weeks in that I was told lithium could start working. But the lithium pills hadn't begun fully working. I think that day I understood exactly where I was in life.

A lot of thinking about the past few years began to take place I was trying to make sense of it all, talking to old friends and asking them why they left me and what changes they had seen me experience—things like that.

Accepting the fact I had bipolar disorder came quite easily to me, beside the few bumps in the road. But the road never does seem to be completely smooth wherever you go.

The story of my diagnoses went like this. My mom picked me up after I jumped in the fountain at school and was suspended. (That's another story. Just pretend you know the story for now. We will get to it for sure later.) We fought in the car, which was the norm in those days. Then, finally, she whipped the car around and said she was taking me to the psychiatric hospital. I pounded on the dashboard and demanded her not to and that it was unnecessary. But we arrived there anyways. My mom told the people at the front counter of the hospital she thought I had bipolar disorder. They assessed me. And at the time, I was bipolar, but I wasn't psychotic enough to be institutionalized. I did need extreme help though.

I still didn't think I was bipolar at the time, so when they put me in the office that was supposed to be a waiting room until the doctor came to see me, I reorganized all the plants and magazines, trying to seem crazier. This was all a joke to me. I couldn't believe I was there. I spoke with the doctor, and it actually felt kind of good because I hadn't spoken to anyone about problems I had been having for a long time. But they had seen no need to keep me overnight, and my mom was strongly encouraged by the doctor to take me to see a psychiatrist.

Once things settled down a bit, I believe my mom told me what I'm about to tell you now (or maybe it was after my first visit to the psychiatrist that she told me). But she told me a little bit about bipolar disorder and why she thought I had it, which made me feel a whole lot better.

My mom had known something was up with me for a while now; she just didn't know what. Then, finally, a young couple from the church, friends of my mom, told my mom they thought I had bipolar disorder. Their son had it too, and I was showing a lot of the same signs.

She must have seen me worshipping at church. I would sing, get really into it, and then fall down and not have energy to get up. And I'm sure I let an uneasy feeling off in the room that I think I let off at high school in the church. But most of the people at church (whether they were just well behaved at church or all the time) didn't give me hard time; most of them were really nice to me. Not to say I was always doing something completely wacko. The incident when I fell down only the people in the row could see me, and they thought I was just praying, which I was—mostly praying to get myself up. Although I was worshipping at church by this point, I still hadn't really gotten into

Jesus. But the pull had begun. When my mom had heard this, she knew immediately that was what it was. My mom had experience working in psychiatric hospitals before and couldn't believe she hadn't thought of it sooner.

So off to the psychiatrist now! We talked it over with him, and he decided, yes, this was bipolar disorder. I described to him a little bit about my life, which happened to show him I had almost all the symptoms of bipolar disorder. I took it pretty well. I really didn't care. I was open to learn about it and see what the heck this thing was. I wasn't like, "Oh yes! This is the answer to all my problems. This is why I have been acting this way!" No. I just looked into the possibility that yes, I might have it. And when I looked into it for myself, I would look in books and on the Internet and read through the symptoms, and then finally, for what felt like the first time in my life, I did some self-evaluating, and I realized, yes, I was experiencing a mental illness called bipolar disorder. Then I looked up some of the cures for it. And they were all medication. Oh, and there was one other one they talked about and that was electroconvulsive therapy, which isn't recommended. So I tried the meds. *What the heck,* I thought.

I was already off marijuana by the time I started taking the meds. Before my diagnosis with bipolar disorder, I smoked marijuana like it was going out of business. I had more smoke going through me than a chimney on a cold Christmas. It was awful. Later on, we will hear more about how smoking marijuana made my illness worse and what traumatic life events marijuana led me to. I had to get off it—that was the deal with the doctor—before I was allowed to go on meds. I was off when he told me that. I had made my own decision by then, but after a month or so on meds, the agitation was killing me, and, foolishly, I got back on for a bit; then I got off again for good. You're not supposed to be on any drugs or alcohol while taking the meds. It screws them up. What really happens is drugs "act on brain chemicals that first stimulate, then over stimulate, and then ultimately destroy the brain's fragile relationship to mood. The person then becomes more uneven and experiences even more mood changes."[2]

A large percentage of people with bipolar disorder also suffer from alcohol or drug abuse. They self-treat themselves. "Snorting cocaine will give someone in depression an intoxicating lift. And a stiff drink can be calming to someone who is agitated."[3] Marijuana will do the same things. While these self-treatment methods may work at first, helping you feel a release from your pain, it's actually only making your mood swings worse and your chemical imbalance even more imbalanced. Giving your brain drugs—depending on which drug—if it's cocaine, it's like playing on the teeter-totter with the weight of the world on the other side; your mood is always up. And if you play with some other drugs, more sedating ones, it's like playing on the teeter-totter by yourself; you stay real low. Then, once the drugs wear off and the damage has been done to your brain, your moods go back and forth like you're playing on the teeter-totter with someone the same weight and you're fighting to see if you can be the one up. So while one side of you is pushing to go up, the other side of you comes crashing down and you're back and forth a lot.

So this is what I'm trying to say. My initial reaction to bipolar disorder was to go on meds. Maybe me and the other guy on the other side of the teeter-totter could just chill and be an even balance. Although those weren't my thoughts at the time, they were more desperate, more like: "Fix me!" You also have to remember if the meds don't fix you right up, you have to take some responsibility. There is a slight chance they will fix you up right away or at least clear up a lot of your symptoms, leaving you with leftover ones you must overcome. Medication is manmade; it makes mistakes and is not perfect. But the power of the Lord is divine. He will and can heal you if you believe.

How Does the Lord Heal?

- Overnight?
- Through medication?
- Over a few years?
- Never?

I learned he does whatever he wants. When you trust him, he will do what's best for you! What I learned is what's best for me isn't always my plan. But as I get closer to him, my plan becomes his plan and I am closer to being on the same page.

# IF YOU KEEP TRYING, YOU WILL NOTICE CHANGE

To give hope, I have selected a few stories or incidents that will show how I noticed a direct difference in myself after a whole year of medication, hard work, obeying my morals, and just plain keeping my head above water.

Before I start my story off, I would like to comment that there's something about being bipolar and being disconnected from people that can really affect you. That effect is you seem to not be aware of what people may be actually thinking. It may seem harsh to say there may be people not understanding what other people are thinking. And maybe it is, but there's something about being disconnected to the point of not even knowing what others are talking about that makes life wrong.

For example, last year when my bipolar disorder was clearly worse and things were close to out of hand.

I remember being in the same predicament I was in today. That predicament was—and maybe you can relate—that my family and I were late for *church.* I was ready. So was my brother, Dale, but Mom was still getting ready.

Last year, I would walk in the house from outside where I was waiting and yell, "Come on. We're going to be late." This would stress everyone out, but I could never figure out why. I thought I was just motivating everyone to hurry up. It seemed like they were all just sitting around, not talking to each other, and slowly taking their time while getting ready. But really they were trying to hustle their butts off to get to church on time, and when they heard me yell, "Let's hurry up. We're going to be late," it came off as if I were angry and if they didn't hurry I was going to be even angrier, and I had proven in the past that when I'm angry, I can be really scary, unfortunately. It was not a good scene.

This year, I came in the house. My instinct was to yell, "Come on. We're going to be late." But I didn't, and I just walked through the house, and when I looked at the clock, I gasped for air. I think they heard me because they said, "Hair, hurry and straighten." Then something happened that I started to notice: these people (my family) were already in such a rush, and they didn't need me yelling. Last year, I just never noticed that they were actually concerned about being late. It's as if I had gotten out of my own head and begun looking at other people.

I was sixteen or seventeen when bipolar symptoms really showed up strong in my life. A year or so after I had been diagnosed with bipolar disorder, I had this "whatever" attitude. I didn't care about anything. This would make my dad furious. You can see the direct correlation in the improvement in my relationship with my dad when I started caring about things and when I didn't. Like the old proverb says, "A wise man hears his father's instruction," (Proverbs 13:1). "A person who heeds correction is sensible," (Proverbs 15:5). "A wise son brings his father joy," (Proverbs 15:20). Why not bring your father joy? Suppose your father has wronged you, maybe even hit you. You're in a rough predicament now, because you cannot be wise without bringing him joy. But be wise and put the hurt aside because he won't be the only one you bring joy to. You will bring joy to your mom too. That relationship didn't work out either, you say? Well, I am one hundred percent positive that if you're wise you will bring joy to someone. So do it! Shoot for the stars! Hold nothing back!

A big step for me to have started caring for my life was getting off marijuana. So by the time I had started really caring for my life again, I was on meds for my bipolar disorder and off marijuana. I started cleaning the house, taking care of myself. I started going for long runs, sometimes seventeen kilometers at a time. I had to slow the running down though because my knee started to hurt. I tried to do a triathlon one day. At this point, I was still suffering from mad depression, irritability to the point that cars driving by would make me mad, and deep insecurity was not helping the issue. Before I tell you why and how I did finish that triathlon, let me give you some insight on what I had to go through in my fight to care for myself. You will see how my exercise of choice, in this case, doing triathlons helped conquer some of the symptoms I was facing from bipolar disorder that were trying to pull me down.

I had to fight to stay awake in the afternoon. The depression was so bad all I wanted to do was sleep. I was reading the Bible at the time, and I read some verses like these on laziness: "Lazy hands make a man poor, but diligent hands bring wealth," (Proverbs 10:4). "Anyone too lazy to cook will starve, but a hard worker is a valuable treasure," (Proverbs 12:27). "The sluggard buries his hand in the dish; he is too lazy to bring it back to his mouth," (Proverbs 26:15). "If a man is lazy, the rafters sag; if his hands are idle, the house leaks," (Ecclesiastes 10:18). "You lazy people can learn by watching an anthill," (Proverbs 6:6). "Having a lazy person on the job is like a mouth full of vinegar or smoke in your eyes," (Prov.10:26). "Work hard, and you will be a leader; be lazy, and you will end up a slave," (Proverbs 12:24). "Being lazy is like walking in a thorn patch, but everyone who does right walks on a smooth road," (Proverbs 15:19). "Being lazy is no different from being a troublemaker," (Proverbs 18:9). "If you are lazy and sleep your time away, you will starve," (Proverbs 19:15). "If you want too much and are too lazy to work, it could be fatal," (Proverbs 21:25). "Don't be so lazy that you say, 'If I go to work, a lion will eat me,'(Proverbs 22:13). "A door turns on its hinges, but a lazy person just turns over in bed," (Proverbs 26:14). "A lazy person says, 'I am smarter than everyone else,'" (Proverbs 26:16).

So every time I slept and then woke up in the morning and wanted to go back to bed, I would think of these verses and feel really lazy as I lay in my bed. And don't get me wrong I had to work at it. I would meditate on those verses as I lay in bed, sometimes, and still fall asleep. Now, when you're bipolar, depending on how far you have come in the recovery process, you do need to take it easy and stay away from stress. So, sometimes when I napped, I didn't feel so bad, but other times my conscience was on me. I found a lot of the reason I would feel so tired was because nothing was stimulating my mind, the mind that felt slowed down from my psychosis. So that's why I picked up running.

I always did like running. That's why every day I chose to run seven kilometers, and then I eventually worked up to do a triathlon. Well, I was a few kilometers shy in the biking and running area, but I knew I could do it. It was just that my knee started to hurt. I believed God was telling me, "Yes, get physical exercise, but, dude, it's not your thing to be running these triathlons." Which I respected. So I just ran a few kilometers every day and played basketball. I started to feel more like Paul, the way he felt about being a Christian. His motivation to be a follower of Jesus went kind of like this:

> Everyone who competes in the games goes into strict training. They do it to get a crown that will not last; but we do it to get a crown that will last forever.
>
> 1 Corinthians 9:25

Don't get me wrong. This running business was painful. It didn't come easy forcing myself out of bed every day to *run.* It was one thing getting out of bed. My mind was like, *You got to be crazy thinking you're going to go running now.*

I kept running for exercise; it's good for the health. Running definitely had its ups and downs for me. It had its up and downs during the process of the actual run, but overall it had one up: it was benefiting my health, and I was outside getting fresh air, all while learning discipline and how to persevere through hard times.

I remember being in seventh or eighth grade and running these distances and getting that burn you get in the chest and cramps, but there's something about running when you are going though *all* the bipolar symptoms that makes running that much more strenuous. Not to mention you feel like dying.

I look back and laugh at how, even during running, I could see my moods going up and down throughout the run like I mentioned earlier. One stretch of the run I had full energy and would run with large, paced-out strides and smell the air through my nostrils and enjoy every bit of it while hearing the birds chirp. Then I would turn the corner, and I was almost crying the pain was so intense, the birds chirping were hurting my ears ... *Just keep breathing,* I would tell myself. And my thoughts would flood all throughout my head, and they would make me want to stop, but I kept going. Then, there I was again, feeling a bit better. Things were a bit more bearable. If you noticed, I explained the urge to stop running coming from my thoughts. When I first wrote this chapter, I hadn't realized one thing I have now learned about bipolar disorder that you truly need to know and do. We need to be like Paul and the other Christians in the Bible who lived by this line Paul wrote: "We take every thought to make it obedient to Christ," (2 Corinthians 10:5). Bipolar disorder seems to flood you with so many thoughts that weigh you down it feels like the sky is raining nails and razor blades that are piercing your skin and hurting you emotionally and mentally. I understand that everybody goes through difficult thoughts, and I completely empathize with that. Even a runner's mind needs to stay strong in order to keep on running. I understand that. I have been there before. It's tough. Then there's bipolar disorder. It's a lot different. Proof of that is the fact that I have always run long distances before. I just always have. I even broke a record in eighth grade once for a long-distance race. That doesn't matter, though. That just proves that, yes, I can do long distances. When I described my thoughts weighing me down and making me want to stop, I was only 300 meters away from my house. It already felt like flames were burning through me. That's why continuing was so difficult. But it can be done, and things will loosen up for you. There isn't anything you can't handle.

> God is faithful; he will not let you be tempted beyond what you can bear. But when you are tempted, he will also provide a way out so that you can stand up under it.
>
> 1 Corinthians 10:13

Maybe this story will help you understand where pain comes from. I had been told this story some time last year. One morning, a woman was spotted doubled up in pain and moaning and sobbing. When asked what was wrong, she responded, "I don't have physical pain. It's the pain of the thoughts I'm having that is doing this to me." Turns out this lady had bipolar disorder.

The more I have taken captive my thoughts and corrected lies in my head and turned them into truths—truths I have found in the Bible—the more healing that has come my way.

# WHY DO BIPOLAR PEOPLE GET SUCH INTENSE THOUGHTS THAT ALMOST SEEM UNBEARABLE TO HANDLE?

The answer is, I don't know. No one knows. My opinion on it is that our unbearable thoughts can be used to benefit us. I have spent nights thinking of nothing except all the disaster and devastations of the world. These thoughts brought me to great lows in my life. They also created compassion in me that I now have the opportunity to use for good. The thoughts showed me the reality of the world we live in. It gave me purpose in life. It gave me direction. It definitely showed me all the areas this life needs help. Erasing child slavery, feeding and housing homeless, decreasing sexual and physical abuse rates, lowering divorce rates, decreasing prostitution or eliminating it, helping crack addicts recover from crack, helping people sober up from alcohol and other drugs, and stopping senseless war are all things that need to be done.

When you ask the doctors why people get bipolar disorder, they have their theories. In the 1960s, bipolar disorder was thought to be rooted in psychological trauma. Psychological trauma could be caused by anything ranging from bad parenting, sexual abuse, physical abuse, seeing the death of your parents, etc. To cure those, all that was needed was some good psychotherapy. That was the solution to bipolar disorder.

While that theory still stands, it is like a chair tipped on two legs, ready to fall and become a distant memory. Although I think it will always play a part in the search for the cure or cause of bipolar disorder, it has now been replaced with faulty body chemistry being the cause of bipolar disorder.

This theory came about when medication was given to bipolar people and they were almost instantly relieved of their illness—which would be pretty darn good medication if it fixed the problems of your past. Most scientist, psychologist, and psychiatrist would agree that bipolar is a faulty body chemistry.

Now that they know Bipolar is in the body chemistry, they are searching in the genes. They believe there is a relationship between genes and environment, which can be very true, because I find that a bipolar person's symptoms can often be triggered with stress, thus starting with genes and then being affected by the environment. It hasn't been completely ruled out, but it's not very likely that bipolar disorder would be brought on entirely by environment. My reasoning behind this is that bipolar disorder seems to be seen at certain ages, eighteen to twenty-two and thirty to forty, or people have it the day they are born. Their environment may affect—almost certainly does affect—the severity of ones symptoms.

Some people with bipolar have bipolar in their family history. Studies show that a person with bipolar is "two to three times likelier than someone without that family history to have bipolar disorder."[4] This shows that genetics seem to have a huge role with the onset of bipolar disorder. Family trees are usually checked by psychiatrists if a person is experiencing symptoms of bipolar disorder. Sometimes, Bipolar is confused with other mental illnesses, such as unipolar depression, reactive depression, schizophrenia, and schizoaffective disorder. If a psychiatrist is leaning toward a diagnosis of bipolar disorder, he or she will become more confident with that decision if there has been family history of bipolar disorder.

# KNOWING THE DIFFERENCE

One common thing schizophrenics have with bipolar people is a sudden race of thoughts and a very high rate of speech, almost sounding like a tape in fast forward. Remember those? They have a little strip of film on them, and they play in tape decks. Well, fast forward one of those, and that would be an extreme case of someone with rapid speech. The difference between the bipolar person and the schizophrenic is, if you listen closely while the bipolar disorder person is talking, he jumps in and out of ideas, but he comes back to his main point, while a schizophrenic is impossible to keep up with. Or I have found another form of rapid speech; I'd call it conservative rapid speech. No doctor has talked about this, but I found that if a person is aware of their rapid speech, they may try and contain it and not talk at all. Possibly laughing would be their way of talking, where they would laugh hysterically because they were bursting with energy but did not want to just go on rambling. They felt like they needed to scream, but they wouldn't, so they hold it in. It may create anger. Yes, I believe there's a way to turn that energy into something positive and let it come out a different way other than rapid speech, and that would definitely be laughter. Or you can look at it the other way. What's wrong with talking fast?

# IMAGINE A WORLD OF HOPE

If you really want to get into theories about environments affecting bipolar disorder, we can. Let's consider it for a chapter. Why have you not simulated the idea that we live in such a fast-paced environment that a bipolar disorder person is simply a portrayal of the society we have created. Everything bad society has done or is doing has accumulated into an illness called bipolar disorder, let's say. That is the patients' burden, their burden alone. They have taken on what society has told them to be and are taking it to the extreme. For example, sexual promiscuity is a way of life in the club scene. Now you have bipolar disorder, which has a symptom called hyper-sexualization. Bipolar people often find themselves with many strangers. Women can be attracted to bipolar men because they let off such a strong sexual aura. Maybe I'm more of a conservative Christian on the subject of sex, as I have chosen to wait until marriage until I have sex. Part of bipolar is I'm attacked by this hyper-sexualized symptom that I have, and it causes me to feel extreme sexual energy that you should not normally feel toward a lot of females, thus making it harder to stay pure. Many men may experience hyper sexuality even though they do not have bipolar. For me I have gone through times of normal sexual tension between women that I was attracted to. There have been other times where this tension flooded upon more women any man could handle, even King Solomon, and made the day almost unbearable. As God has began his work in me he has began taking hyper sexuality away from me. There is a difference between hyper sexuality and normal male sexuality; one is much more extreme than the other. But what if the environment has caused bipolar disorder? What about the society that loves danger and violence? With every film made that has some form of violence in it, we feast on it. We absolutely love it as a society; yet, in real life, if it's done, we look down upon it. How many incidents have there been where bipolar people have gone what some people call "bipolar on someone"? And it is despised, looked down on, and a stigma is even given to all bipolar people. (The stigma being they're all violent.) Just like people who dress in all black; they all cut their wrists, right? No. Here's another one. The advertising industry has gone absolutely nuts, advertising everything they can imagine. From tampons to expensive trucks, they all have fancy advertising. While on the other hand, people with bipolar disorder get labeled as having symptoms such as going on "manic spending sprees." We're everything this society wants. We give you violence. We buy your materials. We talk fast so we don't have to waste time that is so precious to you, and we sometimes fall in to the temptation to participate in your sexual promiscuity because of hyper-sexualization. What is wrong here? What is the problem? Shouldn't you be happy? Why then have you locked us in cells and put us through electro shock therapy in the 1930s? That didn't stop us until the medication came around. I don't want to get too ridiculous, but the government paying us a thousand dollars to keep us off the street so we can barely live—that's if we had no job of course—is all right. But shouldn't you instead be changing the way society is? Haven't things gone too far, so far that you have to do nothing? Are we so far in over our heads that we can't even see what direction we're going? Has so much piled up that even our high-power bulldozers can't even barge through? Have we given up hope in everything we do? Can we start to remember we need to shoot for the stars? Can we give up despair so that we can complete the dreams we have? Is all lost, or have you found it? Because once you start marching in the right direction, you have nothing to lose and only all to gain. We need hope, planet earth. We need hope.

**We have spotted it, Captain. It's on the X chromosome.**

As bizarre and minimal as this may seem, research was conducted on two families, and each member who had color blindness also had bipolar disorder. This was much too rare. No way was this just a coincidence. "The researchers concluded that the gene for color blindness, which is located at the bottom of the X chromosome, must be very near a gene for manic depression."[5] Knowing this makes sense to researchers. They now know why it's not often passed down from male to son as much: because men only have one X chromosome while women have two.

# WHICH BIPOLAR DISORDER ARE YOU? OR, FOR CURIOSITY'S SAKE, HERE ARE THE DIFFERENT TYPES OF BIPOLAR DISORDER.

### Bipolar I

People with Bipolar I are the people with bipolar disorder that usually have the best stories to tell. Doctors and researchers acquaint this type of bipolar disorder with people doing the most "outrageous things,"[6] and "outlandish things."[7] And, to a point, they're right.

Once a person gets fixed up on medication or uses a strong sense of morals to differ from what's right and wrong, they can conquer even the toughest situations. For example, they may start believing sex is wrong before marriage, and believing that firmly may stop them when they get a euphoric high and their sex drive goes through the roof while their energy captivates many women, and they have the desire to have sex with all of them, to *actually* have sex with all of them. We will get into how morals can save you from tough situations later. Right now, I want to share some stories that bipolar people have done in the past that are sometimes unheard of.

On average, Bipolar I people have highs and lows that last for three months at a time. There is an interesting story of a man who went into a very long-term manic episode that is very rare for how long it lasted, which was four years. He began to feel that he was "charged with saving civilization from famine. For years, he hoarded cans of food in his basement from floor to ceiling, until there wasn't an inch of space left."[8]

There are stories of men and women who start to hallucinate and see terrible things or think extreme things. I have a friend who thought he was God. He literally thought he was God. He was the most innocent man I have ever met, but when he called the police and told them he was God, he hung up the phone. Next thing he knows, he has the SWAT team at his house yelling, "Put down the phone." He yelled, "But I am God." He tells me that story with a little smirk. He knows now that, obviously, that was crazy, but he didn't catch it at the time. What's there to do but laugh now? He didn't remember all the details of the story, but I guess he was a bit more aggressive with his words then what he thought, so the cops told him.

Countless people, while going through a manic episode, have stayed up for whole weeks, even two, without any sleep at all. During this time, they aren't just doing nothing. They're going full-fledge into activity all day, and as you may have already perceived, yes, they almost kill themselves from exhaustion.

I have heard of bipolar men becoming so manic while causing crime at the same time, and when police officers tried to take them down, it could take up to seven officers to take one man down, and even that would be a struggle for the officers.

One of the biggest things a Bipolar I person will do is go on incredible spending sprees. They will buy three new cars, a new house maybe. There's even a story of a rich man who had bipolar disorder who paid random people on the street to be his servants.

Being spontaneous to the max is exactly what a Bipolar I person would be. Patty Duke, when she was younger, in a manic episode, tells the story of her finding some guy and getting married that same day.

Often, a Bipolar I person's thoughts might blow through the roof, and they will have hundreds of thoughts, giving them hundreds of ideas, and think they can complete all of them in one day. The funny part is they do sometimes. I have been like this before, although I didn't feel out of control because, at this time, I knew I had bipolar disorder and was able to notice, *Yes, I am having a flight of ideas.* But I just said,

*What the heck! Let's try to complete them.* It wasn't anything that was going to harm anyone. Once, I just got up and almost sprinted 10k. Surprisingly, I didn't feel much pain the next day. I jotted down crazy notes. I just wrote as fast as I could think, and the writing was so messy. I also worked at school work at an incredible pace and then went about town on my bike and did what seemed a million small activities, swam, ran, jumped, and just plain worked my butt off.

I think the worse thing I did that might have classified me as a Bipolar I person was when I had bipolar disorder for about a year and was on no medication, plus I was on marijuana, self-treating myself—not knowing that I was, but I was. I got it in my head that my girlfriend at the time was cheating on me. She went to a different school than me, and it was about 2km or so away. It was pouring rain out, but I was so certain that she had cheated on me or was cheating on me at that second. And I needed to confront her. I was devastated. I felt as if it had actually happened. So you can imagine what my girlfriend thought as she was running from a portable to go inside with her binder over her head, because of the rain, looked over to see what was supposed to be her heroic boyfriend, sprinting through the field soaking wet with what I bet looked like a look of despair and defeat all over his face, yelling out "Why?" She was like "What?" I believe there were people walking by her who just gave me a weird look and kept on walking, but I didn't care. I was so devastated. Then we talked it over, and she couldn't believe that I would think that. She was mad at me, of course, and I'm sure a little freaked out, but I sort of blamed it on a girl in my class who told me I was right; she was cheating on me. What made the girl in my class say this was this crazy theory I had—I can't think of it right now, but it was bogus—and the girl who sat next to me said, "She definitely is cheating on you!" She said this because she was convinced of my theory. And for some reason, I completely believed her. I figured, *girls know girls. She must be right.* If that is not the biggest episode I had that may help classify me as Bipolar I, it was certainly up there in the list of biggest things that would help classify me as Bipolar I.

You see, I was Bipolar I at one point. I never thought I was God, but I was defiantly heading that way. Getting off of marijuana and getting on meds and applying my morals to my life helped a lot, and I'll talk a bit more about the stages of Bipolar I have been through once I explain to you more about the different types of bipolar disorder.

Another story of a lady with Bipolar I going through a very emotional high time is "Fifty-four-year-old Marjorie says she would have a hundred ideas and feel that she could implement everyone of them—write a movie script, paint an entire apartment in one day. She'd call friends at six o'clock in the morning and talk non-stop, just because she was up and feeling vigorous. 'I would do a lot of physical things like moving all the furniture, cooking for an army, polishing all the silver.'[9] Marjorie said."

In a full-blown psychotic mania, a person loses grip on reality. When a person with Bipolar I comes out of their manic state, they drop into a depression that can be disabling. That's why it's nice that the government gives disability paychecks to people with bipolar disorder. But, oops, that's another thing we're getting into later. Their mood will drop so low that they spend days, weeks, and even months facedown in bed, not being able to move—maybe to go to the bathroom and possibly eat, but not much.

You see, my medication didn't work right away. It has been a long process so far for two years, and they still haven't seemed to fix it all. That's why I have other ways of coping, like building a strong foundation of Christian faith under me that can hold me up whenever I fall.

When I first started taking medication, I had dropped out of school after a bit of a manic episode. After that *episode,* we will call it, I guess you can say I *came crashing down.* I was in my bed for a few months straight. I got out of bed to go to the bathroom. That's it. Maybe sneak a drink or snack, but nothing big. I would just lie in bed and not move. I didn't care! At that time, the walls were fascinating enough for me. The angle of the roof was enough to think about. I just didn't want to move. I could have stayed there another year, but I decided to get up and do something. And I might as well share now that I got up and built a shed. We had some old wood in the back, and my dad would work until 3:00 p.m. or so. During that time I just built, my body hated it, but my soul needed it, so I kept doing it. As much as I felt I hated it, building the shed was actually fun; but it was strenuous because, I think, at that point of my life, I was more irritable than ever before. The sound of my own hammer annoyed me. The dog next door barking annoyed me even more. Every bark pierced my skin. What I hated was the irritability. I thought I was going to have a heart attack.

Unluckily, the old wood had some old nails in it. So I had to take all of them out, and, oddly enough, I would get irritable and angry at my irritability and be so depressed. So I didn't have much energy to do anything about my anger, but with what energy I had, I ripped those stupid nails out for hours, until I was driving myself nuts. Looking back, it was if I was talking to a demon inside of me—*If you're not going to let me have fun, you're not having fun either*—and then I began working my butt off. Good, hard work will drive any evil away. Running makes the lungs better. Whiteout covers a mistake. Good always conquers evil in the end.

When most people drop into these lows, it's common for them to have no sex drive, attempt suicide, lose hope, have no self-esteem, feel slowed down, and simply enjoy absolutely nothing. . I would like to say if you are experiencing that form of depression and you have been for a while, I think there comes a point when you have to simply just tell yourself, *Wow! This is fun.* At least set a bar and try. Sounds ridiculous, I know, but it's amazing how much taking captive of your thoughts will do for your life. It turns it around just a little bit more. Sometimes truth comes before feeling.

## Bipolar II

Normally, Bipolar II does not have the high highs of Bipolar I, but it still has the very low lows. "They have recurrent depressions, but without the psychotic manic episodes; instead they experience brief 'hypomanic' (less than manic) episodes."[10] The person with Bipolar II in a manic stage will feel very euphoric, extremely energetic, and possibly very excited.

I recently read that people have been speculating that in a number of sales, people go into a hypomanic state. There have been stories of Bipolar II people while in a hypomanic state selling double or triple the amount of cars they normally sell. This isn't to say all salespeople are hypomanic, but there is that speculation out there.

A Bipolar II person, like said earlier, can have periods of disabling depression. People with this will cry for days on end. One lady described her depression through a painting where she drew her interpretation of the flames of hell with a woman carrying her head on a stick in front of the flames. The lady said how she felt: "detached as though I didn't know where my head was."[11]

Dr. Askikal says:

> They can accomplish a lot, and even though they take risks and sometimes act impulsively, they are charming and intense. They generate a sense of excitement; people catch their highs and tend to like them.[12]

It is said that because of the Bipolar II energy when in a hypomanic state, they can be extremely fun to have at parties. Any place where there are a lot of people and their high energy is accepted is where they are great to have around. Not to mention that the productivity rate that they, without relinquish, demonstrate in jobs can be very useful to the subject himself and his or her employer.

## The Cyclothymiacs

Cyclothymania is a subgroup of bipolar disorder with weaker highs and lows than those typically seen in Bipolar I or II. Cyclothymaniacs have high and low cycles that last only three to five days, bouncing back and forth between high and low a lot faster then Bipolar I or II.

One of the authors of *Brilliant Madness,* Gloria Honchman, delicately elaborates, saying, "They start something with great enthusiasm and don't complete it." [13] I think we all relate to starting something with great enthusiasm and not completing it. Why is this crucial evidence to diagnose someone with bipolar disorder? Or, better yet, why are they starting and not finishing? Upon pondering this question, I have come up with a few theories that could be true. First, I started with examining myself. What better way than to study bipolar disorder when one has it himself and can have personal insight, rather than looking at something through a microscope. I don't need a closer look. What I see is what it is; it's firsthand.

I found one reason I have started something with great enthusiasm before and did not want to finish it. It was because I was thrilled at the new adventure and this new adventure stimulated my mind, so I attacked it and went at it; then the work became strenuous, and the thrill of starting something new wasn't there anymore. When one gets to this point, a decision has to be made. Do I continue and display a strong work ethic and finish this project, or do I find something that will stimulate my mind again so I can feel better? A few projections can be made for why I want to stimulate myself. First, because why wouldn't I? And second, to be more elaborate, because life is too difficult when I'm not stimulated and depressed. Not stimulating my mind means possibly dropping into depression. Third, it feels so nice to be stimulated, energized, and focused on something, even if it is a short time that I'm focused on it.

I'm going to argue that this problem, while I completely agree may be harder to conquer than an average college student's procrastination—due to the depression, manic states, and constant battle of the mind—can be defeated, if not with medication, then with self-control and determination.

The theory that a bipolar cyclothymese starts projects with great enthusiasm but does not finish is a great to look at while starting to pinpoint whether or not the subject has cyclothymese bipolar disorder or not. If you find out they do, can you please tell them first that the problem they are facing, and or a cycle they may have started, is starting with great enthusiasm and finishing not at all their tasks. Then remind them—actually, *tell* them—they have a choice. Say, "You can finish your task. It may be hard, but you can do it." Encourage them.

When I hear a story like the one I am about to reveal to you, that I had read from Patty Duke and Gloria Hochman's *A Brilliant Madness*... Well, first of all, before I go any further, I was deeply impressed by this book. I am not here to insult the book whatsoever. I just need to comment on a few things from it. There is a story of a young woman who would rent an apartment, furnish it with passion and joy, and then she would find some reason to move on. Her excuses were the view was less than she expected. The neighbors were noisy. She was tired of peach and gray. She preferred a loft.

Now, I'm not saying this lady does not have bipolar disorder, but do you know what else I see in this lady? I see someone searching for stability. Can I get an amen? Later in the story, her parents wrote her off as a *drifter.* That isn't family. That is just sharing the same genes. The lady needs Jesus, and if she wants to give me a call, she can. No one should be cast off as a drifter. If someone is searching around them for stability, the stability they need is the stability within. For where there is struggle, Jesus will come. He says to his people, "Come to me, all of you who are weary and burdened, and I will give you rest," (Mathew 11:27–29). Go to Jesus; ask him to give you what you need inside to be stable... ask for him.

There have been complaints that a bipolar person could not pursue his or her dreams. If that is true, it is because he has lost hope in this world. Hope makes any dream possible in any situation. "You can do all things through Christ who strengthens you," (Philippians 4:13).

### Rapid Cycler

A rapid cycler's mood changes from month to month and day to day. They change so fast the two moods will run into each other. The moods change so quickly men and women experiencing this will actually feel like they are going to die. I have been there before. I was a rapid cycler at some points in my life. We will talk later about what exactly I was, but with moods colliding, it will leave you feeling like you're going to die. So if you hear someone you suspect is bipolar, take them serious when they say they feel like they're dying. They may not be exaggerating.

Clifford Whiiting Beers laments in his autobiography *A Mind That Found Himself* about the very problem of not being taking serious.

> To relatives I said little about my state of health, beyond the general statement that I had never felt worse—a statement which, when made by a neurasthenic, means much, but proves little.[14]

# HOPE THROUGH THE SAVIOR

I name my chapter title this solely because I have been to a place where I could do nothing. My dreams were big, but I could not reach them at the present time. How could I pursue a career that involved a lot of communication when I could not properly communicate to a single soul on the planet at that present time? If I had not received hope by putting my trust in God, there would be no point of marching forward. Hope made me realize what I was doing right that second was what was needed for my dream to be complete. I had hope that I would be better. How? Because I had faith. Hope surrounds you and takes a load off of your life.

# MY DIAGNOSIS

When bipolar disorder really showed itself in my life, I believe I was in grade eleven, but it might have started in grade ten. You could tell because I started hanging around a different group of people. And through reflection on my life from now till then, I started acting weirder. By that, I mean I did different things then normal and started smoking pot more heavily.

I had not yet dropped in into a very low low or really high high, at this point, but definite change had taken place. It wasn't until grade twelve and the end of grade eleven when I started to experience more Bipolar I symptoms. The girlfriend episode; the countless hours spent just laying in the grass, letting my elated thoughts take me away to some other world; and I began break dancing.... Now, break dancing was not a bad thing, but dancing excessively can be a sign of bipolar disorder, especially when one is manic. The breakup with the girlfriend seemed to kill me. It wasn't just her though. It was everything. Everything was going away, and I didn't even notice it. The depression probably wasn't a result of the break-up with her; it was just the natural path my life had to go through.

What was going on? I was way to into marijuana, my body began slouching a lot my mind felt more slow than it has ever felt in my entire life. I remember walking down the halls, and all I would notice was one movement of a head turning slightly left and that thought would stick in my head till I got to the end of the hall so all I noticed was a head move here and a head move there. Nothing else was happening in my world. Becoming manic, I would do manic things, but my manic episodes were never too extreme but maybe just enough to be considered Bipolar I. Jumping in the school fountain (which I talk about later), experiences I had at the clubs break dancing, and the way I perceived the world around me all were things that may classify me as Bipolar I. An example of the way I perceived things was when my imagination had gone through the roof while I was throwing javelin. There were times I imagined it all to be like the movie *Troy* when I was at track meets. There were times I would camp in my tent like the main character and be alone and not say a word, not a word to anyone until I threw my javelin. When it came time to throw, I would let out a monster yell and throw as far as I could and then walk away with no expression, showing no emotion.

My imagination going wild also had something to do with me accusing my girlfriend in the stormy rain that she was cheating on me.

One time, I went into such a blank stare while driving, I ran right into the back of a BMW. Thank goodness the owner didn't make me pay for it. I would have been in huge debt. This was, of course, when things were worse for me. I would not agree with a law that said bipolar disorder people can't drive, but if one who is at his worst, where I was at the time, it might be a good idea not to drive.

Not only did I show extreme symptoms of bipolar disorder, I had become disgustingly sinful, that everything I viewed was evil. My mind sickened me. I can't believe God would save a wretch like me.

I didn't have to be confined to the solitary cell in prison to be alone in this world. I already secluded myself. When I did go out, I remember once being at a party, and some guy for no reason tried to attack me. I had no clue why he was doing it. On a different night, he attacked me again with a knife. Being in the place I was at the time, not knowing what was going on around me, incredibly confused to the point that I hadn't a clue what planet earth was like, I quickly tried to figure out what was going on while he walked toward me and I walked backward. A guy named Ryan jumped in and told the guy attacking me to leave me alone, which was a good thing, because I was still trying to figure out what was going on—and not just why he was mad, but what the heck was going on in this world, why I was feeling that way. I left the party, but my ride was still at the party, and no way was I going in looking for him. So I walked a distance away from the party and hid under pine trees while I watched the party. I kept feeling all these different types of energy levels coming off of everyone from the party, and the screams they made at the party, you know the party screams: *woo.* Those *woos* scared the crap out of me. My nerves were on edge.

I remember when things were getting real bad just before I dropped out of school. I was standing in a hall, with people I barely knew, and I kept falling to the left. I would just start falling that way while the people I was with had such a look of concern over their faces and asked, "Are you okay?" "Yes. I'm fine," I would reply. But I darn right knew I wasn't, but I couldn't figure it out. I guess I was happy when they diagnosed me with bipolar disorder; it gave me a place to start thinking. I started slowly putting my sinful ways away and transforming my mind so that it would be pleasing to Jesus. That encouraged my bipolar disorder to get better as well.

As I got better, I was more like a Bipolar II with rapid cycling. But I seemed to have a grip on things and never did outrageous things or things I was unaware of. Speaking of unaware, I should share a story with you my mom told me the other day. In grade twelve or so—I don't remember this at all, but I should—I took all my mom's patio stones and ripped them all up as if I were looking for something underneath. My mom was too afraid to tell me to stop, even though she just did so much work putting them in, because the look I had on my face was so intense that she didn't know what I would do if she interrupted me. This was when I was bipolar I.

One of the biggest things that killed me was the drop in my self-esteem. I'm starting to make eye contact with people more, and it feels great when I do. It actually feels like people listen to me when I say something. That's the only thing that really bugs me—my communication—but I feel it is coming back, and I'll be so happy when it does because God is great. Every day, a new mile is walked, and the more I keep walking, the brighter everything is getting. People who knew me during my rough times tell me they can't believe how much better I'm doing. I appreciate their encouragement.

Okay. Let's back up a bit here. I said I am more of a Bipolar II now. My reason in saying this is I seem to have a grip on things, which still, in my personal opinion, stand true, and I don't find myself doing outrageous things like being unaware of full elapses of an hour at a time. But yet I show one huge sign of Bipolar I that we talked about earlier, and that is staying manic for a long period of time. Maybe there should be new diagnoses. I have seen what you call manic in me all summer—racing thoughts, alert, usually quite energized—but I still feel like crap. You can pay attention to your mood as hard as you want, but it's impossible to track completely because, like a person without bipolar disorder, my mood to changes under the circumstance. Waking up in the morning, and me being more of a night person, I feel low when I wake up naturally. Now, I don't know if you normally feel like death in the morning and don't want to get up, but I do. What is feeling like death? Feeling like death to me is when you beg at the feet of God or someone to take it all away because it is all feeling too unbearable. But you get up anyways and still feel useless, but as soon as you start an activity, your what you would call manic signs appear. You can just feel it in your face, this energy piercing through you, and your head is working so fast your brain is trying to expand out your ears. But if Dad comes by and starts a conversation, I reply, we talk, and if he wasn't my dad, I bet he wouldn't know I had bipolar disorder.

I can feel pointless and weary and useless at the same time as being manic. Okay. So you call this mixed state. Which is mixed state, so if I haven't already established that, yes, I do suffer from mixed states. I am able to agree with that because while I'm depressed, I feel manic. I feel depressed, agitated, and get really bummed out, but at the same time, I'm having racing thoughts and irritability that could be associated both with depression and manic states.

So now the real truth I have to search within myself is am I really down to a Bipolar II, or am I actually a Bipolar I mixed-state rapid cycler? I lean to want to call it Bipolar II because it's less severe and makes me feel like I have gotten somewhere. And I have certainly gotten somewhere. Functioning is just part of life now, whereas before, it wasn't. Why then do I maybe want to call myself Bipolar I but feel I am not anymore? Well, maybe because I have for so long dealt with seeing things in the corner of my eye that aren't actually there. I'm used to it. We have all done it before. You thought you saw something, and you whipped your head over to check, and that something actually wasn't there. I have done that, and it happens quite often, usually when I'm alone, not all the time though. One incident I can recount closer to the date I write this was one day on a nice bike ride home down a country road, it happened three or four times that I thought I saw a giant frog jumping out of the grass. The image I saw was real enough for me to look and get ready and even lightly already start to jerk in the other direction. What I had seen in the corner of my eye wasn't there. I took a deep breath and kept breathing. I wouldn't call it hallucinations though, which would for sure classify me as Bipolar I. Never have I looked at something that wasn't actually there and stared it in the eye and admired its shape, color, and texture before. No, I don't call it a hallucination. I call it more of an extremely strong imagination. The object I saw while driving on the country road was an eight-inch-high frog. The grass beside where I thought I saw the frog was one foot high. The grass and the frog were almost the exact same color. My analysis of it all is, with my nerves on such edge and my imagination and creativity already running rampant, it just created something, but once I looked over to see if it was real, my logic had kicked in; it wasn't real. Most times, when these experiences happen, it is when I'm in deep, deep thought and my mind has driven a hole into a series of questions, which are hooked onto a rope and pulled to the bottom of the ocean, and before snapping out of the deepest thought man can ever go into—at least for me anyway (I cannot account for all men's thoughts, but the thoughts ran deep into the night sky—and then something will snap me out of it and usually make me mad or scare me because I was so happy with my concentration so thick into the thought I was pondering. The something is usually a person's voice that gets my attention and, at other time's, it's the blurry mess of color that surrounds me that I have blocked out, catching my attention with an inanimate object that has formed into looking like something else, like the grass almost looking like a frog.

The best way I can describe this is the vision you get when you stare into a colorful mind illusions book and an object comes out at you in 3-D.

It's not as bad as you think really. It probably sounds worse than it really is. You can't comprehend what I'm trying to describe. I can feel it already. You're thinking, *Woo! That must be freaky!* Because you picturing yourself riding a bike while this giant toad leaps up at you and makes you fall off your bike. It's more like an annoying thing. You know it's not there; then you look, and, sure enough, it's not, but you have to look anyways to double check. Just annoying really.

This happens less than you think too. It's never been anything of a large object either. It's exactly what you go through already when you see a person and then you look and they weren't there and then you get excited and say, "Oh, I thought I saw such and such." You name their name and laugh, and it's no big deal, just like that. My guess is it just happens to me a bit more. Not a lot, just a bit.

What should really scare you is the intense imagination, one that if I were to look out the window, like I'm doing right now, and see a building, I could picture a man falling from it flat on his face, and as he hits the ground, I could feel the impact shudder through my skin. Those negative thoughts must be gotten rid of.

When you run and jump, it sets off nerves in your body and creates senses. Mine already feel set off.

That's why when I imagine myself jumping through this library, doing front flips and back flips, I can feel it in my skin as I imagine it.

In conclusion, it's a fine line whether I'm Bipolar I or II, definitely mixed state and definitely a rapid cycler, and while I never seem to lose control like other Bipolar I people describe it, I do have long spurts of being manic; but at the same time I'm depressed, so I don't usually have defined high and low times. I always just feel the same. If I drop into a three-month depression and have no manic symptoms within a few months, then I will know for sure that I am Bipolar I. But even when I am manic, I do still feel more in a mixed state. All in all, over time, I have slowly been getting better or I have just learned how to manage myself more. Either or both are good, and God is awesome.

# DEALING WITH THE FAMILY

It's said that, because of the intense energy and then the sudden spellbinding lows in people with especially Bipolar II but any bipolar disorder person, they can be hard to live with. This is before medication, of course, or maybe even after depending on the success of the medication. When a person is unaware of having his or her illness, this may make things worse. I think that being aware of what you have and the symptoms you are experiencing are huge steps to overcoming your illness. We're going to talk more about that in our next chapter. There's a lot you can do to be a better family member than anyone you know if you try hard. Let's face it. With doctors out there saying in all their books basically that it is hard for bipolar people to live with family or even have relationships, the odds are against bipolar people, and the thing is they're right. It can be hard. It takes time and patience to get through. Also, a lot of encouragement helps. Try it! Encourage your family. Treat others as you would like to be treated.

If you live that principle out, things will go your way. Maybe not right away, but they will.

Picture this. Your friends or family came and just gave you a massage. After they do that, try asking them if they would like a neck rub. Have something you work on, your own little project that keeps you busy, something you can do to be productive. If there is ever a family dispute that you can't handle in the state you are in, then the activity you have chosen—whether it be building a shed, working on the car, drawing a picture, painting, writing, Web site designing, exercise, you name it—if it's healthy and only benefiting you and others around you, do it.

Let's face it. Your family isn't going to be there to meet *all* your needs. They can't possibly fulfill everything you need, and they are going to disappoint you. In my home, whenever there are problems going on and I feel like everyone is being insensitive to my needs and *that they just don't understand me* or if the whole household has gone crazy and everyone is only thinking of themselves, thus not allowing anything to work, before I make action and try to fix it—which, if I do try, it makes things worse at times because I'm not doing it right—I just leave the house and pray to God, knowing that there's somebody always there who can be relaxed and ready to listen. Knowing this keeps me alive. When I'm at my wit's end and I hate everything and I'm just sick of life, God's there, just chilling, and I listen, or if he doesn't say much, at least I can talk to him. He will work it out when problems are to big for me, which, they will be for you. There will be problems that you cannot handle, just so life-sucking, brain-squeezing, fluorescent light bulb-smashing over your head, annoying, tough, hard problems. You have to give them to God. What other choice do you have? He's offering you peace if you come to him. He promises heaven after death if you do come to him. All you have to do to come to him is hear what he says, and all he says sometimes is, "I sent a Son down to you. He was ridiculed, beaten, and crucified. Do you believe me?" It's not difficult. It's not brain-squeezing. The florescent light bulb stays in the garbage or socket where it belongs rather than a delinquent teen pulling it out and popping you over the head with it. The idea that he died for us is soothing—well, maybe tough, and hard, depending on how much you want to debate over it—but it's certainly there, and all I'm saying is try accepting the truth. If you don't like it, it's not like you have signed a contract stating you cannot turn away.

If you're where I was or worse or even better and were worse before and then better or just anyone in some type of problem—which means all of you—you know what I'm talking about when I say, "Where do I go from here? What am I supposed to do now? This sucks. Why can't my family get along? Where is the love?" If anyone is going through these questions, they need Jesus.

## BEING ALERT AND AWARE

They say knowledge is power. In the case of bipolar disorder, it is. It can give you that power over your illness. Understanding and knowing your symptoms and which bipolar disorder you are can help you overcome your illness. Like I said, you cannot completely rely on medication to completely cure you. If it does, great, but don't rely on it 100 percent in case it doesn't work.

What do I mean by being aware? I mean understand that if you feel that anger coming on, figure out ways to calm it before it escalates. Read, go for a walk, breathe, do something. Learn what you can do when you drop into a low so you're not completely disabled. If it's hard to get around and do things or if, because of your lack of focus, you find it hard to organize things, then write. That is what I do. Or, study and go to school. That's what I do also. And you also have to keep trying. Even in my lowest low, where I could not socialize with anyone because I could barely talk, I was able to read and write, which gave me some kind of purpose until I came more out of depression. Maybe sports are your thing, but I guarantee, if you think long and hard enough, you will find something that will keep you occupied and give you a purpose-driven life until you can function and do more things.

Even while you're real low, try and enjoy life again by doing an activity you can do. Maybe it's sewing scarves, slippers, or hats for the winter time when it's cold, depending on the part of the world that you live in. Maybe you can make them for friends and family. Maybe you can play sports; throw a ball around; and even though it's not even enjoyable because you feel so low, you can practice aiming it really good and throwing it really hard, and you will see yourself improve, and you will see your skill level improving. Then this will lift your spirit a bit. Next thing you know, you're enjoying it.

Even if you don't enjoy your activity right away, it's still nice to do. Wouldn't it be nice to have made slippers, hats, and scarves for your whole family, all while they were away? What a surprise that would be. Or your friends or maybe just some needy people? They could possible be very proud of your efforts, despite what was going on. I would. I would be proud of you. And if there is no one to be proud of you, God is always there for you, and he's proud of hard work. I guarantee it.

In my grade twelve year of high school, despite the drugs and the lows that brought me incredibly low, to the point teachers were worried I was going to commit suicide ... Yes, I haven't told you yet, but my teachers told me that a little while after they thought what they thought. Nonetheless, they told me I looked like I was going to commit suicide. They said just the way I walked and sat looked as if I wanted to kill myself, and they were terribly concerned. That was nice of them. Seriously, it was nice to be concerned. But thank goodness I didn't or even try. I don't think I was even thinking about it at that time because I didn't even realize I was depressed at the time. How I felt was just life for me in my head.

Anyways, despite all of that, I joined the track team and picked up javelin. I was extremely depressed while doing it, but determined to beat the school record. I had never thrown javelin before, so I had a lot of learning to do. I threw javelin all season. I traveled to all the track meets, and I threw 35 meters on average, which was pretty good. It was getting me top six at the track meets, but the school record was 39 meters. I had to beat it. Just throwing the javelin and watching it soar threw the air and then poke right in the ground and then getting it again became a routine for me. I just did it. Never really excited, I just did it because I had a goal and I wanted to complete it. Eventually, coming out to the field and throwing my javelin became the great release of the day. It began to be a bit better than the rest of the day. I began to enjoy it just a little bit because I had focused my mind on it and never gave up. The rest of my day wasn't like that, so something was set apart. I enjoyed something. Then came the final track meet of the year. Everything I worked for had to be done. I needed to throw over 39 meters. My first throw was only 36 meters. My second throw, I took off from the start line focused. I trotted up the runway and then began picking up speed. I looked straight at the field, ended with my three-side stride routine that gave me all the extra boost I needed, let out the largest yell as I threw, and bam. The javelin poked right in the ground. There was a gasp in the crowd. I didn't know why. It looked like a normal throw for me anyways. I almost had stepped over the line, so I backed up, waiting for the measurement to come in. With all the life in me, which wasn't much, I celebrated with a simple smile toward my mother, who had been watching, when the announcer announced I had thrown 50 meters. I had beaten the school record and received a nick name: the ten-meter wonder—not to mention all the bigger guys were furious with me. They thought for sure they had a chance to go to the Ontario's championship , but only the top two go, and they knew who first place was. It was the guy who was a professional javelin thrower who has javelin shoes, a javelin outfit, and everything. So there was one spot open for them, and that was second. There were about three of them who would always battle for second and could usually throw around 42 meters. So they tried their luck, and nope. Sorry guys. They didn't get to go on.

That's why I know you can do something while you're really depressed. You just have to set your mind on it and practice hard. Overcoming adversity is all about building character. Even if I didn't make that throw, I wouldn't have cared—probably because I didn't have enough life in me to care. But I don't think I would have cared if I did anyways, because all year I tried, and all year I received the glory you get when you overcome something hard in your life, a sense of peace maybe, a sense of encouragement, whatever it is that comes rolling and gives you an immense lift in life, that helps you move forward, move forward just like my javelin did—sometimes a meter and then sometimes[15] meters—depending on the plan laid out for you in your life.

# DREAMS

Keep dreaming. If your life is straight and you're doing great things for yourself, you're putting yourself in a position to dream dreams that will come true.

One dream of mine came true. Since grade seven, I played basketball. I was never the best on the school teams. Street ball was a bit different. I seemed a bit better, but it was never my calling to be a professional basketball player. I was a short player and got good at those teardrop shots. Before a lot of my bipolar disorder symptoms appeared visibly but started to show up quite minor, I was on the high school basketball team and I was a sixth man kind of guy. Then, after basketball, the only thing I cared about was smoking pot and going to clubs, the all-age ones.

Then came the time when I was diagnosed with bipolar disorder. I went for my runs I was telling you about earlier during that time. I also started playing basketball in my driveway again. I had a gravel driveway, but that didn't stop me. You could still do lay-ups, and shoot the ball. Working on your dribbles was hard, but thankfully, most my life that's all I worked on. Shooting was what I needed most practice with. So I started playing basketball every day. I mean, come on. I had dropped out of school, had no close friends at the moment, and put a few hours every day into correspondence to get my diploma. I had time on my hands, man, and I had gotten rid of the drugs, and I was battling laziness, but when I kicked laziness right in the butt, I had time, man. I had time.

So I would shoot 'em every day. I started getting curious with my results so I would take one hundred three-pointers a day. I had a three-point line roughly marked out. It was twenty feet away, and I would set goals for myself to beat my score.

And you know those racing thoughts you get if you're bipolar? Well, I took all those thoughts while I played basketball and imagined up a goal for myself. I would graduate from high school doing correspondence and play college basketball at whatever college I went to. Bam! Sunk it again! Bam! There's another one! Bam! I started making it more interesting. I would always keep track of how many consecutive shots I could make every day. My dream had begun. It was always there, since grade six, when I said I would play basketball in college. But now I was determined, and there's one thing I know about a man when he's determined: he can do anything. "I can do all things through Christ who strengthens me," is what I tell myself every day (Philippians 4:13). My mom showed me that verse when I was in grade six or so. It remains my life verse, something that helps me when I want to give up because I believe it to be true. After shooting hoops and carrying out the rest of my day, I would go to sleep, and then I would wake up and do it all over again.

Maybe you're a morning person, or maybe you were a morning person and now you're not ever since you got bipolar disorder? "Err," I would groan as I tried getting out of bed. *I know it's so hard to get up out of bed when your feeling bad.* I emphasized. *I don't want to!* my brain screamed as I tried crawling out of bed. Then, once again, I remembered those verses on laziness. I got up, wandered around the house, trying to think of something I needed to do or something to look forward to, something that would make myself feel a little better. *Because shooting hoops, running, stretching, doing my homework doesn't seem like anything I want to do right now,* I thought. *I know they are what I should be doing,* I would reason. Then I would reason and argue with myself, *Once I do my activities, it usually feels good and gives me a chance to let me forget about this pain. I should do them. But I want to sleep,* my fleshly desires fought back to say. Then I thought, *Well, I'll take a shower. Showers feel good.* And I would begin to *ease* myself in to the morning.

It's important for me to give myself some credit at this point. I have gotten off the pot, alcohol, I'm trying to do school, and I'm trying really hard to be a better family member. I was trying hard to be a better person period. Yet, when I got in the shower, I began to worry. *I don't want to waste water. Poor people could use this water,* my mind cried. Then I was stopped right there and told by what felt to be God saying, *I am a God who gives grace. I love the homeless and needy people more then you. They will be taken care of. Right now, I want to take care of you. Right now, I want you to be blessed with a hot shower.* I thought, *Well, it does sound like something God would say. Maybe he really is trying to tell me that.* I would then let the hot water soak my body. I also felt like God did not just want me to take a hot shower and not enjoy it. I felt he wanted me to enjoy the hot shower and love it and count it as his blessing.

I got out of the shower and felt the heavy burden of transition of changing activities, and the transition wore me down. *Okay. I should do homework now or go for that run. I want to care for my life,* I thought. But all I was imagining was passing out on that bed of mine and forgetting about everything. *Have a bowl of cereal! Enjoy it! And try not to feel guilty about it. Then, if you still can't get yourself motivated, I'm going to have to say it—suck it up. Just start running. Do something. It will help. Trust me. Start doing your work. Just do it! Do it, man! Do it!* was what seemed God was whispering to me. So I had the bowl of cereal and completed all the goals I had for that day. It took some of God's divine intervention, but he certainly pulled through for me.

I did make it to college, by the way. I even played basketball. My shooting percentage wasn't half as good as it was in the driveway. There's something about six-foot-something monsters jumping in your face that makes it a little harder to score. Overall, it was fun though. I got through my first year of college with great grades, and the team finished sixth in basketball. I also met a great group of guys that I will mention to you over and over again. They were that great! Thanks, guys! And Coach too! Thanks!

# BIPOLAR MISSION STATEMENT

Bipolar people need to gain self-control. I have to cross my arms too hard in defense of bipolar disorder. Don't get me wrong. I have had my times of giving truth to the definition of the stigma of bipolar disorder. But, man, today and every time I talked to someone about bipolar disorder, they would first tell me they didn't know much about it and then they would go on to tell me a story about, in this case, a friend's boyfriend who went crazy obsessive over her and it resulted in himself overdosing on pills. (The boyfriend was bipolar.) His ex-girlfriend by now became aware of the overdose through a text message from him, and she called the police. They found him passed out in his room. Luckily, his life was saved, but only to leave more harassing phone calls to his ex-girlfriend. I constantly am hearing stories like this after asking random individuals, "What do you know about bipolar disorder?" They usually recite a story they know of someone who had bipolar disorder, and that is all they know.

Our goal is to change this, people! Our goal is to give bipolar people a good reputation. And this is how we do it. We exploit ourselves for who we really are! When someone is asked, "What is bipolar disorder?" I want to see a glee come across their faces. I want them to remember the person they met who was bipolar and although sympathy runs through their hearts for the immense pain and sorrow a bipolar person carries, he or she will remember how cool, exciting, new, and fresh they were. I want them to remember the gift they have been given from the bipolar person who by adding an exciting twist to their life because his or her energy encouraged them. I want them to remember the interesting view he or she had on the world which will magnify the visions and thoughts of the one with the memories. The love shining out of someone with bipolar disorder, despite the sorrow they feel, is breathtaking and drowns the one witnessing the love with more love. Glory on high. Thank you, Lord, for your glorious being. Help people walk together because we need each other. People need you, Lord, and I understand you want us. Together, victory and the crown of life can be ours, people of this earth, whether you have bipolar disorder or not.

# THE OVERCOMER

I find this saying to be a great saying: "It was all worth it." Hopefully, your life goes a way where you get a chance to go through a rough part of life and come out of it saying, "It was all worth it." I hope that on everyone. I also hope on everyone no rough parts at all. But sometimes it seems they're inevitable. But if there are rough times, I hope they're all worth it in the end for everybody.

Eventually, people will learn to realize that suffering can only make them better. Pain is gain. You have heard it in sporting events, but I live to tell everyone it is true. No matter how bad the pain is, people will eventually gain something positive out of it. Even the death of a family member brings more insight and wisdom on the topic of death, which you can share with others.

Maybe some people have endured the pains that seem to come with life and their dreams have all come true and more are in the process of becoming real life?

They may have learned so much from every bad fall they had. And they did get up, and they kept trying again. They didn't give up! They are an overcomer! Congratulations! Keep going! Don't be prideful once you have overcome; stay humble like you were when you felt like nothing.

Give, give, and give, and let others give to you. Hold captive all your thoughts and you will be fine. Thirst for love, and may your heart quench for hope. Keep loving and hope will come chasing. With faith, it can all come true.

For those who have overcome, say hello to victory for me. Don't bother turning back to say goodbye. Just leave. Flee from what holds you back, enjoy your food, take delight in the scenery, and let people carry you. Soon, you may have to carry them.

Let knowledge and wisdom latch on to your sides, and they will never let you go. Be thankful for peace. Ask for it, if you don't have it, and it will be yours. We all deserve peace. It starts with all of us. If we all live our lives peacefully, we all will, in return, give peace to the next person, and peace will spread in place of disease.

> Love is patient, love is kind. It does not envy, it does not boast, it is not proud. It is not rude, it is not self-seeking, it is not easily angered, it keeps no record of wrongs. Love does not delight in

> evil but rejoices with the truth. It always protects, always trust, always hopes, always perseveres.
>
> 1 Corinthians 13:4–7

Living in love promotes peace. Living in love helps you overcome.

# MORALS: YOUR SWORD IN THE BATTLE

Once I got on medication, I still had many symptoms, and one symptom that came out was my anger. I think humans, whether they believe in God or not, have a moral guideline that says, *Do not hit, yell, or break things.* Some of them, of course, have a stronger moral code then others. Regardless, society has told humans it's illegal to hit in every country, I think. Society also tells a human yelling is inappropriate and breaking things can lead to vandalism. Those are good things society has taught if you ask me. The stronger our belief that hitting is wrong, the harder it is going to be to let our anger take control and hit. If you were taught by your parents at a young age not to hit, it will be even easier for you to not hit. If you were never taught such things and possibly have seen those things go on in your home, instilling those morals in you with strength that will hold will be harder but can be done. Your heart must be open, and you must really believe it is wrong, so much that if you do hit you will feel ashamed of yourself, shame that will put you in line so you can be a better person.

I think if you're bipolar and you are reading this and you suffer from irritability at some point during your illness, which almost everyone seems to, you have to have a strong belief that what is making you irritable is not doing so on purpose. Whether it is a person or a machine, if you believe *they* or *it* is doing what they're doing on purpose to irritate you, it will lead you to more anger and more insanity. If you believe strongly that they are not doing it on purpose, you can begin to look at yourself and figure out techniques that will make you less irritable. Sometimes, just looking away and looking back will clear your head, maybe turning up the radio a tad if you're in the car, breathing defiantly helps, and possibly talking it out with someone—especially if you really don't believe that person isn't out to get you, but something keeps telling you they are. Ask, "Are you trying to bug me?" They may reply, "No." Then say, "Didn't think so."

# LEARNING FROM THOSE AA MEETINGS

What's the first step of anyone who has ever been to an Alcoholics Anonymous meeting? Admitting that you have a problem! We can learn from this technique. The same holds true to all our situations. If you have a problem, which we all do, admitting it makes it a lot easier to deal with. It diminishes the problem and puts the problem back in its place. It's now a problem that you're ready to deal with. The problem is no longer you. It isn't a monster that is unbearable.

If I'm paranoid and I start fretting about the problem in my head and never come to terms with the problem, I will never get anywhere. As soon as I say, "I'm all paranoid about..." And say it with a half smile too, then I recognize, *I just have to work on that. Just because I get paranoid sometimes does not mean that symptom controls me. I'm just aware of it, and I'll make it through.* It's amazing when you do the right thing and feel like you're doing the right thing, how much the right thing is actually helping you. Yes, you admitted you were paranoid about an event in life that came across your path. You also admit you're feeling a bit shaky about admitting that. Everything in you wants to cover it up and give in to what the paranoia wants—maybe drinking, smoking, or getting angry and breaking things. You feel that what you're doing isn't working because you don't see immediate effects and it hasn't taken away the pain. Yet, what is constructive in your life will begin to grow while you leave your fear behind.

# MUSIC

Don't be afraid to sing a little tune aloud. Praises or tunes can bring ease to your soul. Before the anger bursts out, let it come out peacefully. Sing a song. I recommend singing anything that is on your heart, but guard your hearts and watch your tongues because they have the ability to set forest fires (James 3:5).

I believe that God created me, and I believe a lot of our purpose is to praise him. I sing praises to the Lord. I just make them up. I usually don't sing straight out of the hymn book. For instance, use key themes like thanking, encouraging, loving, and help me songs. Everyone needs help, everyone needs encouragement, everyone needs love, and everyone needs thanks. Your thanks, love, encouragement, and help me songs can be to people or God or both. These are great things to sing about and have floating through your head, leading you toward peace.

# LOVE WILL FIX IT ALL

Love will fix it all. Medication can only do so much. When love is applied to any sore, it will be healed. Forgiving someone is a form of love, and it heals. For example, if I hurt someone with my words (which I have) and maybe not purposely hurt them, but out of maybe ignorance we will call it, I hurt them. Then, later, I find out I have actually hurt them. For me, it's time to push aside my pride. And in most circumstances, as soon as those simple words, "I'm sorry," come out of my mouth, those wounds can be healed. That is love!

When I get in someone's face and egg them on to hit me because I feel so angry I want someone to feel my anger too and they say, "I will not hit you," and just walk away, this is love.

I'm down and out, depressed out of my mind. A professor picks this up while at student body retreat and sends me home with all the leftovers. Yummy! This is love.

A teammate runs by during a game and says, "You're doing great." This is love.

I'm running. I'm late. The train is about to leave. A stranger holds the door open, thus stopping the train from being aloud to move. I catch it! This is love.

Tense, annoyed, frustrated, out of nowhere, a loving hand gives your shoulders a quick rub. This is love!

I think we have all heard it before. You should be more concerned with what you give than what you take. Except I always tried to run first in line for food as a kid. We're not perfect. Besides that, we all need love. We are always looking for what is best for us, but what we really need is something we can receive, and this is love. Love cannot be forced. Letting someone in front of you, putting them first, will show them love. If someone bursts in front of you without your permission, they may be in front of you, but it was not given to them as a loving gift, and that is what they really need.

Love is medicine. Love is a filter in a dirty pool. It cleans it right out! For it is said that "Love is kind," (1 Corinthians 13:4), and I say love can also be laughter. It is also said that "Love is patient" (1 Corinthians 13:4), for my life, rewinded and played back again, can say this is true.

Love is gentle, love is kind, love is generous, and love is slow to anger. Love is the only beating I enjoy. For when I was not slow to anger, my peers' love swallowed me because they were slow to anger. I had nowhere to run but to feel loved and accepted.

Right now, stop getting angry quickly! Be slow to anger. You're not only doing yourself a favor; you could be opening the eyes of someone else. I remember attending my small group I have been attending for quite sometime now. It was a different format this time. We were having a party and games night. Before we got playing, we were all sitting around. I felt my anger building for no reason at all. Then a girl there asked me if she could move my laptop. I said no, and she did it anyways. I told her to put it back. I spoke to her harshly, an unnecessary harshness.

Than the man beside me, who was also a friend with all of us, said, "Stop speaking to her that way." I foolishly got in his face. Never swearing or saying something too mean, I just used an awful voice, which showed my anger. I was hoping he would punch me. *Maybe it would make me feel better*, I thought. I wasn't about to hit him. I was controlled enough to know better, but I was up in his face, and the whole room was tense. *What am I doing?* "I am not going to hit you!" he said and walked away. I was left standing there, stupid. The party continued. I finally joined in on the fun once I let go of the anger.

Later, feeling humiliated, I apologized to him. This man was my friend. He had spent many weeks in deep discussion in touchy life topics with me; the whole group did. We talked about everything that was on our minds. It was gratifying. I enjoyed it. He didn't hit me. He turned the other cheek. How thankful I am.

Love heals!

# THE NEED FOR COMMUNITY

All I have talked about, love and the stories I have shared, tie in for the need for community. As a person with bipolar disorder, I know how easy it is for someone with it to seclude him or herself. Apparently, bipolar people are not the only ones. This society, with the Internet, TV, iPods, and all has turned into a very secluded society.

The way we travel, in big groups but not talking with each other, the time we spend on the Internet alone in a room—we're always just trying to get alone.

Alone time is good. Don't get me wrong. Even Jesus made sure he got himself to a lonely place where he could spend some time alone, where he usually would pray (Mark 1:35, Matthew 14:23, Luke 6:12). We need to be alone sometimes. Some of us acquire more time alone than others. We all need time alone. Let's just not get carried away.

It's tempting to. It was for me, especially in my grade twelve year, before I got diagnosed with bipolar disorder but clearly had it. During classes, and defiantly during lunch, I would sneak out to the storage shed used for the track and field team and climb up in the rafters and sleep where the high jump mats were just so I could be alone. I usually played Pac-Man on my cell phone or just slept. I was avoiding human contact.

Then, as I got on medication and with God, I started getting around people. I noticed myself; every time a loving situation would arise, I would want to escape, scared. Scared of the emotions? I don't know.

Now that I'm more aware of myself, for me, as an individual, I find that the better the situation is for me, the more I want to escape. Sometimes that comes up with family parties or friends in a big group. My fear tries to take over and get me out of there.

I remember deciding to overcome that fear in one instance, so I walked toward the group of people whom my body wanted to escape from (which happened to be friends and family). I got so incredibly nervous, and then my uncle said something to me, and everyone who he was talking to in that circle turned to me to look for my response. I gave my response; everyone laughed; and all of a sudden, I felt a whole lot better, and then the positive emotions started growing on me.

I know one thing. We humans all get nervous, and it usually happens for us when we go to big events. I guess the only solution is to suck it up and go in hard because if you do, you will have an even better time.

If you're bipolar, you will be surprised with what you have in common with other people. While you may be experiencing a wide spread of bipolar disorder symptoms, another person who does not have bipolar disorder may be experiencing at least one that you have.

This really clicked for me one day after telling a friend about some of my bipolar disorder *problems.* I was telling him about the large depression I fell into when I entered my first year of college and how I would hang around everybody and always feel like it was my turn to talk and then never have anything to say, thus leaving the conversation in a constant loll. One third-year student called us all, the first-year kids, antisocial. That is how bad it got. I just could not talk to anyone. I had a lot to say, but I just couldn't get it out. By second semester, the severe depression left and left me with just depression, and I could finally talk to people better. It seemed like everyone started communicating better. We always had that unity because when one was down, we all came down, it seemed. It's strange how it all worked. After sharing part of the experience I had in college with my friend, he said, "Wow! You sound a lot like me!" Then he shared with me his high school experience. The exact same thing would happen to him, where he would never have anything to say or what he had to say would not come out. He doesn't have bipolar disorder, but we all suffer from a lot of the same things. Use your bipolar disorder as insight, and help people. Use your struggle as a tool for good. Share your knowledge and wisdom.

## DREAM BIG

Sometimes we're given dreams that can give us hope. I speak from experience. Experience is a good friend of mine. He makes whatever I say true to me, allowing you to take it or leave it, in terms of what I say. So, take it or leave it. But I think we can all say when we dream big and chase after that dream. We spend our days fired up more then we have ever been before.

Especially when you're depressed, down in the dumps kind of upset; especially when the depression is for no good reason, I urge you to keep trying. Maybe you're a single mom with a few kids and you just want financial freedom. Maybe you're bipolar, or maybe you're both. Maybe you're young with bipolar disorder and you have big plans for a future career. Keep your dreams close to your heart.

This verse says it all: "Delight yourselves in the Lord and he will give you the desires of you heart" (Psalm 37:4). So far, he has given me some. For example, playing college basketball and just going to college for that matter, and meeting special friends I have met along the way, especially after a few years with not so many.

For me, writing this book was a dream I had, and God, my God, has provided me with an unbelievable amount of motivation that I don't have in the rest of my life to write this book.

Every time a difficulty comes in the day, I take that energy built up from it and write. Some difficulties are quite larger then others. Some still exist and continue fueling me while others have passed by and served their purpose in strengthening me.

What may seem impossible one day is possible the next. You can be delivered from your bondage. While you're living in a dumpster, it's nice to find that fresh apple wrapped in plastic wrap sinking its way toward you at the bottom. Keep finding those apples. What I love is you have made due with the half-eaten chickens thrown your way and held your head high while someone ripped it away from you.

The book *Voices of Reason in Christian History* reads, "We cannot doubt that to this visit we owe the lifelong struggle of Irenaeus against their heresies."15 Irenenaeus did just that; he fought arguments against what he believed. This was his struggle.

If you're bipolar, you already have your struggle. If you want to make use of it, excel at your talent, fight through the struggle. You may already feel like everything is an argument and that waking up is a task, that socializing is difficult. Fight through that, and make a difference. If you can walk those steps, you will receive so much more hope.

I'm writing this assuming that you want to help others. Through your actions, you can. There will be a reward of peace for you if you do. Irenaeus is a famous Christian apologist, and his more in-depth struggle was people kept knocking down his faith. This was at the time of AD 140.

If you feel like everything is an argument, if peace is yet to be with you, then there it is. You, my friends, are enough heroes to me. Actually, right now, you're only a superstar. But now take your talents, your skills, abilities, and gifts, and use them for good despite your difficulty, and then you, my friend, are a hero. Sure, it's not fair, but hey, maybe it is. Maybe it will all be worth in it the end. Find out. Find out with me. It should be an adventure.

If you have already seen doctors and have been taking your medications, and nothing seems to be happening, then what do you do? Feel hopeless? No. Because then you're just giving into one of your possible symptoms.

Is it possible to keep going? Well, hey, what's up? I'm still here—thus far anyways. My religion says I should have a zest for life and be enthusiastic about it. Well, you know what? Half the time, I just drag myself around this place, trying to figure out why I'm dragging myself around this place. But I see the trap already. If I get all upset with myself because I have re-examined my life (another supposed symptom: constantly re-examining your life) and noticed, hey, I'm not being very zestful, and I get more upset and feel even more hopeless with myself because I'm not being zestful the way God wants me to be, then I'm only making things worse. I'm only giving into more symptoms. Symptoms will gang up on you; one will lead you to another. Or I could acknowledge, "Hey, I'm trying! I'm trying to be zestful. I am excited about life. I'm just having a hard time showing it." Or when I wasn't trying, instead of getting upset, I just said, "I can do it!" or I used the Bible verse I really liked. It's one that has been my favorite since I was twelve. I shared it to you already. Philippians 4:13: "I can do all things through Christ who strengthens me." Either way, I wasn't about to fall into that trap, the trap of having one symptom lead to another. At least I was going to *try* not to let it happen. Plus, I believe that *as long as you're trying,* God is applying. The reality is, you're where you're at, and if you don't like it, then you can take it or leave it.

I'm trying! I believe my God loves me wherever I'm at. That's why I like him. That's why I love him. He says seems to say me, "Yes. Show zest in life, even when you're suffering from bipolar disorder, a mental illness. But I understand if the burden you are carrying is weighing you down. It shouldn't be because..." Then he leads me to a Bible verse that says, "Come to me, all you who are weary and burdened, and I will give you rest. Take my yoke upon you and learn from me, for I am gentle and humble in heart, and you will find rest for your souls. For my yoke is easy and my burden is light," (Matthew 11 28–29). For me, he says, "You just need to come to me. I see you are zestful in life, Jason. Others may not, but I do. When you get up with a normal eight hours of sleep and when you spend all day working your butt off, when your body tells you to stop when it normally should be going, and your emotions are going for a roller coaster ride and your brain is in agony and you keep working anyways, I see that you're trying. I will bless you." Now, he hasn't made it clear when these blessings will come or how big they will be, but I feel like they will be big and hopefully come soon. I feel blessed just to breathe, to look at the sky, and to be able to taste. He's blessed me enough already.

For me, loving God and feeling immense pain at the same time can be used as a bonus. There's some kind of inclination I get about God—that when we suffer and don't lose our faith, that he will bless us even more.

I would like to write more to you today, but my chest hurts so bad the anxiety is off the chain. Today, I worked harder than I have worked in a while. I fasted all day, plus built a tree fort for my brother, made a basketball net and screwed it to the shed, and I did a lot of things actually, too many to name. I also got in a huge fight with my brother. I feel awful for it. I guess through all I have done today, I have learned one thing: each activity has something special in store.

For instance, throughout the day, I had to come in the house to call the pharmacy, to explain to them that they had billed me for my medication when I have a drug plan that should cover it 100 percent and should not have been charged at all. All of that is worked out now, thank God.

It was really hard to work up the motivation to call the pharmacy. I was so tired. It was afternoon, late afternoon, to be exact, and that's apparently the worse time for bipolar people who are suffering from their symptoms quite severely—at least it was for me anyways. I also find and hear that for a lot of people, late afternoon is a tiring time. The sun is blazing, you possibly have worked all day, and you're hungry. I felt so low, but dragged myself to call; then I did call, and the lady's voice which I was so familiar with lifted me back up. It reminded me of my relationship I had with the pharmacy and how life still existed outside of the low town of depression. I enjoyed that talk.

Right now, as I write, all I can think about is bed. My arms are tired, my nose is running, I can't think properly, my anxiety is awful. Wait. Maybe this is what the doctor was talking about, overdoing it and such. I guess maybe as a bipolar person, I have to take it easy a bit more then others at this present time.

But I'm so afraid. I'm so afraid of everything for some reason, afraid of life, afraid of living. What is driving this fear? How do I get rid of it? I'm trying to come up with ways in which I could escape and feel better, but I can't think of any. There is nothing. What is nothing, and where is it? Don't even scrutinize and tell me, "Well, if it was nothing, you wouldn't know you were there." I don't want to hear that. I'm sick of arguing—constant battles in my head, me arguing with myself. My thought life is showing in my regular life because that is why I argued with my brother. It hurts. I hate it! I'm sick of it! Then when will it go away? I can't believe other people don't feel this pain. Since bipolar disorder has shown itself at large in my life, I have gained so much understanding of life and gained wisdom I didn't have before, but I also didn't have the pain that seems to come along with it, like being trapped in the desert—the bothersome sun, you can't escape it. If I could just keep the new mind I have but drop the pain, I would be happy.

Oh how nice it would be if every wish I commanded came true in that instant. All I can do is stare at the heavens and patiently wait for the day I will be in a place where a wish wouldn't exist because it would have already come true.

# THOUGHTS OF DEATH

One symptom that bipolar people commonly have is thoughts about death, religion, and the afterlife. I usually hear the term *unusual* thoughts about death, religion, and the afterlife. But what's unusual on this earth, especially when everyone believes a wide variety of things? Is what is unusual just unusual because you don't believe in what the next person believes?

See, what ticks me off is when I hear opinions about this subject, it's always looked on negatively. I think this is one of the more positive symptoms of bipolar disorder. It can be anyways. There comes a time in every man or woman's life where you need to think about these things. Bipolar disorder usually comes in adolescents, or it comes later in the thirties and forties, or maybe you are born with it. Either way, death, religion, and the afterlife need to be looked at, especially looked at in early adolescence. If you have bipolar disorder or if you're depressed and life has been throwing you wrong turns, you will begin to think of these things. Go for it! That's what I have to say to you. Go for it!

Now, there are some precautions you have to take. For example, if you have bipolar disorder or depression or if you're bipolar and going through severe depression, you may be thinking about death but feeling so sad that you think you're deserving of it or you might think of killing yourself. Please don't. People love you. I love you because I love people. If you believe in God, he loves you; if you don't believe in God, he loves you.

I felt suicidal at a point in my life. Here's the story. I moved from Ontario to Calgary so I could attend Alberta Bible College. (They will appreciate that I advertise for them in my book. It truly is a great school.) I had just moved out there, away from my whole family. I had already been on medication for a year now, and I had most of my symptoms still, although they had toned down a bit compared to the previous year. But, man, that move killed me. I didn't realize it, but soon enough, after about three months of living there, I had noticed that I had dropped into the biggest depression I have ever been in. It happened so instantly and without any alarm going off. It just happened, and I lived three months not realizing it. My energy levels dropped. My social skills disappeared. Anxiety and anger were flying off the handle, but so many new things were happening with the move and all, I didn't catch all these symptoms occurring. But then I started to notice it as I reflected on my life. Then a week went by after reflecting, and there I was, sitting on a bench right after drinking chocolate milk and eating a sub. I was thinking about chocolate milk and how I drink it and it goes in me and I just pee it out and how this dumb sub was probably so bad for me and yet I just ate it, barely enjoying the taste, and then swallow and then there it sits in my stomach; then I poop it out. I was thinking how kids in Africa would devour this sub even if it was on the ground in dirt because they're starving. I often thought sad thoughts about kids in Africa. That didn't worry me; those thoughts were good for me. It was my next thoughts that brought upon great alarm.

After I digested the sub, I sat there, staring at the ground, imagining myself cutting my wrist; then I thought about what I was thinking. I immediately told four people from my school, including two teachers. I was never one to think about committing suicide, but how I thought about it so vividly made me think, *I need help.* Talking to those people made me feel better. Then, me being Christian, I prayed to God about it over and over. I didn't stop praying because I didn't want my thoughts to get away on me and actually commit suicide. That's why I like when the Bible talks about taking captive your thoughts (2 Corinthians 10:5). This verse really served me well in my life at that point of time and still does.

The thoughts did go away; the severe depression didn't. Eventually, it did, about two months later. That doesn't mean I still didn't get depressed after that—just not as bad. I think once I got used to the change I was okay. See, when you *just get* bipolar disorder, you're a real sensitive case and everything seems to affect you. I believe that everything affects everybody in some shape, way, or form, but after a psychosis, you become more sensitive. Once you become aware of this, it helps.

It's okay to think thoughts about death. It's good for you because death is real. It happens. Suicidal thoughts you watch out for. But if you venture off and think about death, other than when you're at a funeral that you're going to make happen, you're on your way to making your mind courageous and more understanding of life.

And what happens after death? That's a great question. You need to think about it.

For me, it seems like I rarely thought deeply into these issues until my bipolar disorder fully exposed itself, and now I'm grateful for having the experience of thinking through these things. I still think them through. Some things we will never completely understand, but we can always understand them better.

There's nothing stopping you from freeing your mind from rules on how one should think or act. You can do whatever you want whenever you want. That's free will. Just because we *can* do whatever we want doesn't mean that we *do.*

Don't let yourself think thoughts that are only bringing your character down. You may think of the past and remember how good it was and how different things are now (if you're struggling), and as you think of how good they were, you may get even madder at how things are now; but getting mad at how things are now is only making things before even better, which makes things now even worse.

# GETTING A DOCTOR AND DEALING WITH YOUR DOCTOR

I found a great psychiatrist with his doctorate degree. He was a Christian who was a nice guy. Sometime, we would pray together for the right meds to come. When I first met this doctor, I didn't like him too much. I always got irritated with him. I felt like I never had a chance to say what I wanted to say to him. Once some of my symptoms cleared up, I realized the reason I was mad at him wasn't because of him; it was my symptoms trying to attack me and my relationships again.

How I had realized this was the eight-month interval I had to recover while I was in Calgary, which revealed it to me. Upon return, I went to see my doctor, dreading it, thinking it was going to be annoying and irritable like last time; but I knew I needed my meds, so I went anyways. And just talking to him, I noticed how much my symptoms really had cleared up. I hadn't noticed that until I had gotten back and talked to him. I actually noticed how much they were cleared up with every different person I talked to that I knew before. The conversations were a lot smoother.

### What are simple things you noticed? What was easier?

It was easier for him to prescribe meds to me because I could clearly identify my symptoms. I was having such an easier time voicing my thoughts—and not only voicing them but voicing them clearly.

The year before, I always felt like he just threw me on any med for any darn reason and didn't hear me out. I did go on about nine different meds that year, by the way—or more. I lost count. But I was confused because the communication wasn't there. I didn't know what he was thinking. That year, because I could speak clearly, he was able to speak clearly to me about why he was making the decisions he was making; thus, gaining my confidence in his decision, I felt better. It all started with fixing my problem.

It had a lot do with my communication, it seemed. Why wasn't I communicating well? Possibly because pain inflicts our minds so deeply we are not aware of the world around us but only consumed in what we are thinking and searching our own souls to find a way on how to survive the next moment.

It's been clinically proven that medication helps treat bipolar disorder. It's not a 100 percent, complete cure, but it does help. I figure if the medication isn't going to affect you negatively, why not give it a chance to affect you positively.

I'm also going to note that I am yet to take a medication that changed me overnight or even over a few months. I will also openly and honestly tell you I have heard of very few who have had that success. But it does happen.

My psychiatrist has told me that some of the same medications he gave me, he had given to some of his other bipolar patients. They had helped them within months. I will say yes, maybe over a few months they had helped me, but they never completely cured me. It doesn't mean it won't; it just means it hasn't for a lot of people I have met or heard of and has not for me as well. Seriously, as cut and dry as this sounds, take the pills. Just pop them in every night and morning, depending on the schedule. Never forget. Stay diligent and then let the pills try and do their work. Let them try to give some balance back to your brain. Give them a try. In the meantime, while you're sleeping, chemicals are going through your digestive system, up to your brain, trying to make you saner, more balanced, thus taking away a lot of pain and ongoing frustration. And while you're awake, work hard, and live, and breathe the Word of God, and this will help. If you don't think lessons on how to love your neighbor as yourself and give unto others as you would like them to give to you aren't valuable lessons you need to know in life, then try reading the verses that teach you how to get through suffering throughout the whole Bible, especially the New Testament. Read about Job in the book of Job, and meet a man who truly underwent suffering but somehow held on to God. Read through Acts and the thirteen epistles Paul wrote and meet a man who worked in extensive labor, who was imprisoned many times, was beat down many times, and was near death on more occasions than one would like. Five times he received thirty-nine lashings. He was stoned. He was shipwrecked, spent a day and a night in the depth of the sea, experienced dangers from robbers and dangers from rivers. He spent many sleepless nights with hunger and thirst yet no food. He was cold, lacking clothing (2 Corinthians 11:24–27). Meet Jesus, who died for your sins so you may be forgiven and have eternal life. After you read all that and more, providing your heart is open to learning, you will notice a difference in your life even more, and soon you will be set free from the bondage that holds you down. Don't close the book because you're mad at God. I am a bipolar person. I'm just like you, or maybe you're reading this book because you heard it will help you through whatever struggle you're going through. Either way, this is my story, and this is how I lived it, and this is how it began and continues to grow for me. For me, it all started with Jesus. Maybe for you it hasn't, and that's fine. You can do whatever you like. Anyone can. Don't put this book down because of Jesus. Read on. See if there's something you can find in here that will help you grow and get you through anything you need to get through. We live in a post-modern world they say. We live by stories. That's what I'm told. A story won't hurt you. You, in your heart, have already decided if you want this book to help you or not; so if you, in your heart, are choosing no, I hope there will be some valuable information you can obtain in the meantime. My heart drips tears in hope that the glory God has given us all will be received by us all.

I have taken 1200 mg of lithium for just under two years now, and I have been getting better for that period of time also. I also have been taking 0.5 mg of Risperdal for the same amount of time. That has also been helping me.

I know one thing. I have been recovering. My symptoms have all decreased considerably. Some have vanished. Never have I ever overnight noticed a huge change in me. Through medication or in what I believe God has done in my life, it has been a long-term recovery for me, nothing instantly. It has been like cooking a turkey on a hungry stomach: nice and slow, but very rewarding in the end, wishing you could just stick it in the microwave and zap it in thirty seconds and finally eat it. You may even try and mutilate the turkey while trying to get it in the microwave and leave a mess all over the floor that your grandma kicks your but because of. Then, if you're like me, in the end, you realize there is a certain way for things to occur and you reason that we live in an orderly universe. Things seem to happen for a purpose. But it's all so much to think about in one day, so you just keep on walking, keep on trying, keep looking both ways before crossing the street. Usually, you're just so excited you forget. But it comes down to, "What am I going to live for? What am I going to suffer for? Who is going to be there with me?" You may realize, *I am too weak to do it all myself. I am certainly not a god. If I was, my best trick would be wiping down the table real nice and smooth and maybe vacuuming, and if I am a god, why can I only jump two feet, maybe three if I try? If I'm a god, where's my goddess, and why isn't she helping me clean? If I am a god, I am a god alone, with nothing to boast about, with nothing to boast over. Because the truth is even when I clean, I sometimes miss a spot, and company comes over and finds a dirty cup in the cupboard. How embarrassing is that. I do breathe drink and eat though and take delight in what I see outside, whether it is a clear night sky fluttering with stars or trees dancing in the wind forever and ever, with wonder filling me inside and out until I willingly drown in it. I just enjoy it all.*

I had to go though all these thoughts. As I struggled with my faith with God, I remembered one simple thing. I thought, *The Bible speaks of nature as God's creation for humans. Well, if there is a God, he sure seems to be right about one thing. I do enjoy what I see.*

Sometimes, nothing delights me. I feel despair and sorrow the whole time. Then I met a man named King Solomon in the Bible, who gave me hope. He said, "Grief is better then laughter, for when a face is sad, a heart may be glad," (Ecclesiastes 7:3).

I have been put on more medication during the two years on Risperdal and lithium to see if we can speed up the recovery. As long as the new pills I have been put on don't give me side effects, I'll try them.

Bipolar is a chemical imbalance inside your brain. The medication tries to level that out for you. All lithium is is salt. Its generic name is lithium carbonate, and it is more than just a medication to help set brain levels correctly; it's actually used in fireworks. The deep red you see in fireworks, yes, those are from the mixture of lithium carbonate. Industrial businessmen who pave roads love lithium carbonate because when it's mixed with cement, it dries faster. Lithium carbonate is an odorless, white powder. When you take it, it's released into the central nervous system, where most bipolar people have problems. Then, from there, it interacts by mingling around with a bunch of neurotransmitters. Neurotransmitters are like a bunch of gossipers; they relay information from the neurons to other cells. So, in this case, we like gossipers. The goal is to decrease norepinephrine. Norepinephrine is:

> a stress hormone. Norepinephrine affects parts of the brain where attention and responding actions are controlled. Along with epinephrine, norepinephrine also underlies the fight-or-flight response, directly increasing heart rate, triggering the release of glucose from energy stores, and increasing blood flow to skeletal muscle.[16]

The other part of the goal is to the increase the serotonin levels. With a bipolar person's flight or fight repsonse always activated, it's no wonder they have angry outbursts or try to escape into drugs. But Bipolar is more than that; it's a mood disorder as well, and lithuim is a mood stabilizer.

All doctors put you on different medication. I would suggest suggesting to them lithium first and then going from there. It has the highest success rates. I'm not going to lie. I gained twenty pounds on lithium. I might have lost five since then. Most my life, I had a six pack from the sit-ups I do and the physical strain sports put on my abs. Soccer really works the lower abs, and the twisting in basketball will work the side of your abs while pure sit-ups will give you your bulk. Now, my lower two abs are hard to see because lithium made my stomach bloat. It hasn't bloated quite as bad, but much like the kids from Africa you see on TV, from malnutrition. My stomach has bloated similar to that. It doesn't affect your sport playing though, except you have a bit more weight, which will affect your vertical jump. It may go away. Who knows? (As I edit this book, I already have lost weight, and my stomach has decreased in bloatedness more then the five pounds again.)

Anyways, I would rather see people who have bipolar disorder get off street drugs, stop getting drunk and being violent, and take medication and gain a few pounds than being turned away from a little side effect of medication.

When I stopped drugs and sobered up my mind, this brought me a lot of the way. You have to help yourself. You need to get things on track, learn to live with what you have, be strong because you are strong. You usually don't crawl around when you have legs. If you have strength, use it.

If you are weak, then when you are weak you are strong (2 Corinthians 12:10). Our weaknesses will become our biggest strength. You feel unconfident now? Crowds will soon flourish with your charisma. Nervous now? Bravery will be your alias. Sad and depressed? Soon, you will be someone's sunshine.

Take medication if you need it! And don't say you don't when you do. They can be kind of fun sometimes. One time, I took some medication that didn't sit too well with me; this was one of the worse incidents I had.

The medication was supposed to make me relax so my agitation would go away and bunch of other things, fun things. Well, it made me relaxed all right. Next thing you know, I felt like I was melting. I was all alone when this happened. My dad was at work, and I was at my dad's house that day. I was laughing, but I could barely laugh because my face felt like it was melting. I was way too relaxed.

Then someone called. I picked up the phone. It was for my sister, Amanda, and the girl on the other end was freaking out on me. I think she thought I was playing stupid, but that was the best I could pronounce my words.

And don't worry. The medication was not addictive. I soon felt better and had a nice meal, which tasted very good, seeing how relaxed I was. Then I never took those pills again. I prefer feeling more solid rather than like a candle melting away.

You think that's bad, the worse were these pills. I was discussing with my doctor the name, but I took them so long ago he forgets, and he may have them in records but it's not a big deal. They were some mood stabilizer, I think, and they made me poop nineteen times in one day. I hated those pills.

Lithium is probably helping me, and possibly Risperdal. Although I have my doubts sometimes if Risperdal is even working, but at least lithium has been steady, and I have been improving the way I live, think, and talk. I truly believe God is shaping me through all of this.

Sometimes we need harsh awakenings to wake us up from whatever we shouldn't be doing to get us on to track with what we should be doing. Maybe mine was bipolar disorder. It certainly has woken me up, and I certainly have a better outlook on life now. Just recently, I read a Bible story in the Old Testament about a king who went insane for seven years. When the seven years was up, his sanity was restored along with his authority and power, and he learned to believe in God through those seven years. This is the story of King Nebuchadnezzar.

King Nebuchadnezzar was a content, prosperous king of Babylon. One day, he had a dream. The dream frightened the king, to the point he gathered all the best people in the land to interpret his dream. Finally, Belteshazzar, the chief magician, was the one to give the proper interpretation of his dream.

> You will be driven away from people and will live with the wild animals; you will eat grass like cattle and be drenched with the dew of heaven. Seven times will pass by for you until you acknowledge that the Most High is sovereign over the kingdom of men and gives them to anyone he wishes. The command to leave the stump of the tree with it's roots means that your kingdom will be restored to you when you acknowledge that heaven rules.
>
> Daniel 4:24–26

One whole year later, God followed through with the plan. King Nebuchadnezzar spent seven years in the wilderness, absolutely insane, doing as the dream prophesied he would. When the seven years was up, King Nebuchadnezzar writes this, which is recorded in the Bible for all to read:

> At the end of that time, I, Nebuchadnezzar, raised my eyes toward heaven, and my sanity was restored. Then I praised the Most High; I honored and glorified him who lives forever. His dominion is an eternal dominion; his kingdom endures from generation to generation. All the peoples of the earth are regarded as nothing. He does as he pleases with the powers of heaven and the peoples of the earth. No one can hold back his hand or say to him: What have you done?
>
> Daniel 3: 34–35

It's amazing that a story so close to home for so many mentally ill people is right here in the Old Testament book of Daniel. This story teaches us that there is hope and purpose for everything that happens in life. King Nebuchadnezzar did not go insane for any petty reason. He went insane so he could be a stronger person afterward. Is this story the case for all mentally ill people? This is a big question that I would like to lean toward saying no to. The reason behind disaster varies. It is not always important for us to know why as it is important for us to know where we are in life and be thankful for all things, with trust that God is a great God who is sovereign, acting in love toward us in this great relationship we are in with him.

And like the Christians always say, "God will come in your life and change you and make you a new person, if you let him." I had already given him the permission. I just had my heels in the dirt. What those Christians said came true in my life because my life has seen change at the same time I truly let God change it.

God gives us resources. In this case, for bipolar people or anyone for that matter, he has given us medication. Bipolar disorder, what is it but a mere obstacle one must overcome. If you have bipolar disorder, you can do it. I know you can. Symptoms? We all have symptoms. Bipolar disorder, just crush it with your feet. Hate it. Get sick of it. Crush it.

You feel it? It's all crummy in your chest? Yes, that's anxiety. Half the high schools kids suffer from the same thing. Look straight ahead with determination. Don't give up! Sick and tired? Keep walking! Full of energy? Give someone your shoulder.

Take the pain and turn it to something good. Let it drive you to do something great. It takes guts. Be courageous! Living life constantly feeling confused, not knowing what's happening, only experiencing extreme emotions can leave you feeling lost. But somehow you keep growing, and you keep making sense of your actions through the pain. If this is you I describe, I assure you, clarity is almost there. Giving up is not an option. Be as creative as you possibly can.

Medicine is okay. It helps you. Take it in controlled amounts, and it may benefit you. You won't feel drugged up, woozy, and dizzy, not knowing what's happening from taking medication most the time. The medicine will only work slightly within your brain to a make difference. You won't even feel it happening.

But medicine isn't the answer to all your problems; you have a lot of work to do yourself. I'm sure you're aware of that. Don't be afraid to take medicine because of what others think. Most people are more relived to hear you're on medicine when you're bipolar than anything else.

I usually don't like the subject of medicine because it's like what my uncle says about Christianity. He complains about what I say in my speech. He says, "You give all your achievements to God. You tell everyone it's all him doing the work." I think some people might think the same about medicine. They give everything that happened in their lives to medicine. You have to do your part, and if you do yours right, God will do his. God is always there to help you in every situation. Without the gift of life he gave me, I could not breathe.

But the truth is it is Christ working through me who gives me strength. My uncle is right. Don't sell yourself short of your achievements. You do have to go through a lot. God would want you to feel encouraged. My uncle is an anarchic humanist and does not believe God exists, to put it lightly. So he would want you to take all the credit and give it to yourself. But may I interject and say, humble yourselves and give it to God, your creator. When I am doing anything, I would like to say, thank you God for allowing me to do this. Notice that allowing me is beside a verb phrase "to do" with the adjective *this,* thus meaning you still get credit for doing what *you* have done but at the same time you give it to God, who then gives you more credit for doing what you have done plus giving it to him. He gives you even more credit for acknowledging who "the man" is. By giving it to God, you have put yourself in the hands of a loving God who will never want you to feel useless. So it's a win-win situation. Everyone's happy. Nobody has loss. To think by giving it to God I am taking away from my own achievements and my own power would go against everything Christianity says. But if you are right and God does not exist, would saying, "Thank you, God," really affect me? Because my uncle would say that your entire reality exists inside your own brain. So if my reality is God exists, loves me, wants me, and needs me for the greater good of everything, wouldn't this thought only drive me to greater things, despite if it is real or wrong? The problem with that is that in my reality, I must believe 100 percent that God does exist, created me, and died for me and rose again, so I cannot believe that reality is what you make it. If I believe that I created my own reality, I would be pretty mad at myself right now. How stupid could I be to create a reality that gave me bipolar disorder? Moving on now to try and keep the book on its purpose, and right now its intended purpose is not to stand over the pool dipping toes into anarcho-humanism water. Because right now they have great ideas, but the drain has been pulled and they're all telling me to come to them, but I hear from them that love is selfish. I love you, my uncle. My uncle and I talk and grow together in life. As I wrote this book, this is what he told me. Then I saw him not too long ago and I heard him say stuff about love and it not being selfish. I love the fact we can learn together as find truths in life together as people. It is important never to hold someone to something they say unless he is Jesus because often, that leads to disappointment for yourself and anger for the person who you hold this line to. As people, we all should know that were not perfect.

God gave the doctors the minds to think of medicine to help my bipolar disorder, so I thank him. I also encourage and thank the doctors who came up with these crazy solutions, to help the bipolar brain. I appreciate the time you spent in the laboratory coming up with these medicines. Thank you for giving us something other than a battery and wires hooked up to our brain. Thank you for putting an end to the amount of bipolar people locked in cells because the community didn't want them. Thank you for putting the time and energy into trying. Keep trying. Maybe you will find a 100-percent cure. Then I will thank God, who, in return, if the circumstances are right, will bless you for blessing me, and, everybody, thanks.

I should say one thing. Never force a person you may think has bipolar disorder to take medication. That is wrong. Unless the medication is side effect free and will instantly cure the patient, never do it.

If I was forced to be on medication when I was more ill then I am now, I would have gotten off it as soon as possible when no one was looking. I would possibly have felt bitter toward medication and never have taken it again on my own.

I'm hoping that people just know if you have bipolar disorder or even think you might, go on some medications; seek help; and, most importantly, receive God.

# USE YOUR RESOURCES, AND BE CONTENT

How stupid would it be to have a multiple-outlet extension cord while your fridge and freezer became room temperature all because you didn't want to use the extension cord?

How silly would it be for a politician or a speaker of some sort to pass a bill with his mouth full and without a microphone while announcing issues concerning abortion?

How stupid would it be to have a million dollars given to you so you could enter a NASCAR race and the only stipulation was you had to buy your own car so you bought a moped, and spent the rest of the money on paint to paint the moped, a special acrylic paint, when you really wanted to win the race?

Let's use our resources, people! If medication is available, take it! If people are there to help you, take their help! Let's not burden ourselves like the politician with his mouth full, but swallow, find a microphone, and speak so you can be heard!

You have a voice. You may not think you can be heard, but you can—through books, through anything. The media may be an outlet for you to have your voice heard. The opportunities are endless. We all have a plan. I strongly believe that, and I believe our plans are unique and some people's plans, unfortunately, are devalued.

Check it out. Martin Luther King was not born with the thoughts he came up with when he spoke the "I Have a Dream" speech ever so nicely. He was influenced throughout his life like all of us. Right? Yes!

If he's anything like me, he becomes influenced through the oddest and strangest things and people.

A homeless man on the street walks with me and chats with me, and, through the words he shared, he gave and provided me with insight into the homeless culture and the struggle this world has with homelessness. I am truly thankful for him.

I know people who have no intent of becoming famous, selling books, being on TV, who just want to live a more reserved life and keep to themselves. But they have great ideas. Where would the people you see on TV be without them?

There are people who have a calling to be in front of people while they speak. Then there are people who like to live in the background and not say as much.

Those people inspire the world by inspiring one person at a time. It works because then that one person they inspire then inspires the world. That quiet individual seems to have a louder voice now. It's a truly fantastic phenomenon. Thanks to all who have tried.

It's kind of like the writers who write up plays for Hollywood movies, who are never heard but are behind a lot of genius you see in some films. We all need to be thanked because we all have a part—even though some seem bigger than others, we all do, and we are all a crucial part to the puzzle. Every piece counts. If it were not so, the puzzle would not be complete. I believe my God is a creator who does not make puzzles with missing pieces. I know he is a God of order and intends to make it all fit together.

# BIPOLAR DISORDER, A DEMON

After today, there is no doubt that Bipolar is a demon. If you have bipolar disorder, you are in a one big fight with a demon. All day, constantly, you fight this demon, and it's obvious to the public when he wins a battle.

Today, I will admit what happened. I loss a battle after winning for so long. Today, I gave in, collapsed. I was at a place that seemed to trigger my bipolar disorder the most at this moment, the spot where I'm loved the most: my mom's house. I felt it coming. I needed to leave the house, and I asked my mom to drive me to London so I could go on a walk. But her show was on at eight, and the whole family was watching it together. She said she would take me at nine.

One thing lead to another, and there I was in front of my computer, working on this very book, and my whole body tensed up, and I was tricked to believe that if I was even more tense, I would squeeze all the pain out, so I did. I squeezed. I squeezed hard. And that wasn't enough. I had to make grunting noises to release the pain even more. They were vicious-sounding. By this time, sweat was dripping down my face; judging by the feeling of heat on my face, I was bright red; and I couldn't release it enough. So there I was coughing up what seemed to be my lungs. I sounded sick and disturbed, and I very well was that. I write you this to tell you one thing. Only one thing calmed me down, and that was Jesus.

My family stayed away for a bit during this episode; then my brother came in and said it would be okay. His touch on my back was nice, but not enough to cool me off. He told my mom. She said she would take me right then. What urged her to say this was because I was still once and awhile saying, "Take me," in a very rough voice—my cry of pain, I would like to call it. I thought her taking me would release it all. She finally came in the room and said it would be all right. This did nothing to me. She said a few other things, and they all did nothing for me. Then she did it. She rubbed my back and said, "Sweet lamb of Jesus, bring peace." Everything inside of me loosened up 50 percent. Then my mom told me to just breathe, so I did, and now I was thinking a bit more clearly, and I took the initiative and relaxed myself fully like I could have from the beginning, but now I finally got my bravery back.

It was weird. Something inside of me wanted to act my pain out. I wanted people to truly see how hurt I was inside, what deep turmoil I felt, and by doing that, for me was clenching every muscle I have, and grunting/screaming/coughing at once. The truth is pain is gain, and it creates creativity, and if you harness it, people will truly be blessed by something you have done. Doing what I did was not the answer. What I learned from it was I need more people to pray for me, so if you read this, pray for me. I need all the help I can get.

I wrote the story you just read two months ago. As I go back and edit my book, I find it most important that I add to this topic, the topic being wanting to show people how you feel but can't. I won't say I just discovered it, but I definitely experience it more in full and understood it more last night. What "it" is is finally showing people how I truly feel.

I was in the car with my mom, and for some reason, I always feel the need to show her exactly how I feel. But I'm awful at it. I usually argue with her and get mad at her and, in return, leave her with hurt feelings. I'm so awful at showing my love to her. Deep down inside, I just want to show her I care for her and also explain my pain, but using words never seems to do it. I want to show more of the emotion that is at the center of me. Many people believe it is a sin to be angry or mad, but it's actually not. The Bible says, "In your anger do not sin," (Ephesians 4:26). It does not say, "In your sin, do not sin." Remember, Jesus throws over tables:

> Jesus entered the temple area and drove out all who were buying and selling there. He overturned tables of the money changers and the benches of those selling doves.
>
> Mathew 21:12

He also reclined at the table: "When evening came, Jesus was reclining at the table with the twelve," (Mathew 26:20).

Well, I was not just angry in the car. I was overcome with sorrow and had been for a while now, so the weekend at my mom's went on with arguments here and there and people getting hurt. It wasn't the prettiest sight you ever saw. You would rather watch Niagara Falls dry up than this; trust me. Okay, that's probably a *huge* exaggeration. Niagara is beautiful. But it was not good. Then, finally, on the ride home, we got to yelling at each other again and then, finally, it came. Unfortunately, it took yelling to bring it on, but I cried. And I cried hard. Man, it felt good. I could tell the others in the car how I felt while I balled my eyes out—I mean a gut-clenching, chin-tilted slightly in the air, eyes squeezed shut, fists clenched, and toes curled cry. Tears were pouring, and during the cry, I finally told them what I wanted to say them. It was something that if I were to tell them when I'm not crying, they wouldn't believe because there would be no emotion behind it, even though I would have really meant it. I said, "I'm trying so hard, and it just isn't working." Silence dropped over the car as I said it, and my sister and my mom, who were in the car, finally listened and realized I was trying to survive and I didn't hate them.

The thing I hate about the situation I was in is not the crying. I wish I could cry like that every time I feel that upset without holding it in, but I never can. I contain it too much. I try and release through creativity, so that at least helps, keeps me alive and going. What I hate the most is the badly used anger before the cry, which finally got me to release the anger in a more positive way. And I tell you, crying helps. The uproar of a hysterical cry is sometimes the only way to even come close to how a lot of bipolar disorder people are feeling right now. It doesn't harm anyone, and it releases a lot of stress. I even think that if you're a Christian and trying to become more like Jesus and you do cry, you're being more like him for two reasons. One, quite simply, "Jesus wept," (John 11:45). Two, Jesus said, "I assure you unless you turn from your sins and become as little children, you will never get into the kingdom of heaven" (Matthew18:3). Most children are never afraid to cry.

# WE HAVE FREEDOM

There's good news if you're bipolar in Canada. There are agencies there to help you get on your feet. Plus, psychiatrists are free, and they can prescribe you medication. I lived in Ontario when I first realized I had bipolar disorder. At this point, I had already lost five jobs and working was basically out of the question. Maybe I could make it by working if I pushed as hard as I could, but even then, I think it wouldn't be a job well done to the employer. Besides, I honestly needed that time to recover from my mental illness at least a little bit. Bipolar disorder hits most people around the age of eighteen to twenty-two. What a bad time, eh? At this time, you should be going to college or getting a job and starting to support yourself. Well, I'll give you a couple reasons why there's no need to complain about the timing.

While no time is a good time, let's learn to look at the bright side of things, despite the awful circumstances. Let's enjoy the twinkle of the snow instead of being irritated by the cold breeze blowing at our faces. Let's enjoy the tan instead of complaining about the sweat. Let's enjoy that we have a chair and not say, "But it's too hard."

There are some scenarios this formula can't be applied to. I'm sure McDonald's would say, "Just enjoy the burger, and don't worry about the fat." Or Pepsi might say, "Just drink it up! Enjoy it. Don't think about the calories." Or if you believe in Satan, you know darn right he's saying, "Enjoy the high. Don't worry about the brain cells. Don't worry about the addiction." Of course, they don't say these things directly; they do it in a much more discreet, indirect manner.

While we take a situation that has a good thing in it and a bad thing, make sure it *does* have that one good thing. Don't lie and say that marijuana will take your problems away. I know firsthand that it doesn't. It only made my bipolar disorder worse. Drugs and alcohol often made me feel like I was someone with no thoughts. My only goal when I was on drugs was to find my next place where and how I was going to get high and with whom.

Satan yelled so loudly in my ear, "Get high. Get high. Get high." If I did, I had not escaped anything, It was as if I had run into a wall that said no exit, but I kept trying to run through, and every time I got high that wall would get taller and taller, but sometimes when I got really high and I felt like I was escaping, that wall would disappear; but I was too high and I couldn't get up and move, so I sat there with a bag of potato chips until the wall came back and there was a clear view.

It was like I was a fly making the same mistake over and over. You know how a fly tries to escape through the clean window, but he just can't get through, and he screams, "Bam! Ouch, here we go again. Ouch! Not that time. Let's try again." Over and over, he goes running into the window. I was much like that.

So let's take a look at all the lovely things there are in Canada that can help you with bipolar disorder.

## The Government Actually Will Help You If You're Bipolar in Canada? Whoa! Dude, let's check it out!

I lived in Ontario when I first got bipolar disorder ( like I said earlier), and I needed a time out to try to get a grip on things, but I also needed money, and I also needed an education.

"Well, Jason, you must have been really stuck," you might say. Well, no, because the government in Ontario provides you with a pretty little thing called a disability check. You will need proof from your doctor that you have been diagnosed with bipolar disorder. Then you have to go through an interview and do some paperwork before they can approve you. When they do—and it may take a long time, maybe up to six months or even more—don't ask why they took so long. Well, you can, but don't be ignorant. Just see if you can help the situation any more. Be grateful!

I think the reason for the length in most provinces is the lack of workers and the increasing reality of mental illness. For now, let's give them the benefit of the doubt that they are working hard.

I hope God provides for you while your application is being processed, but when I was accepted, Ontario gave me $750 a month to support myself and 100 percent coverage on my drug plan. (That is only for the drugs that are from Canada. If they are from anywhere else, you may have to pay a percentage.)

So, $750, and if I were to work, I was allowed to make half that before they deducted anything off. When they began to deduct, they would only deduct 50 percent of what I made.

So if I earned, while working, $750, I would have $1300 at the end of the month, including my disability checks. If you're living with your parents, this $750 will be enough to support you. If you're living alone and you're older and you have worked before, you might get workers' compensation or you may have to go to welfare. Either way, this money will provide you enough to support your drug habit if you have one. No! We must not abuse the privilege the government has provided us. People already complain that programs like these enable people and their drug problems. The sad part is it can! It did for me for a month, until I got my act together. Thank God for grace, that I didn't have my money taken away for abusing it like I did. I wasn't disciplined directly by any authority to have my disability money taken away, partly because they didn't know, but I believe I will be judged by all my actions when I die, and that was wrong of me. The point I'm making is that that same money I abused for a month helped give me rest during a difficult time once I got my act together, rest I needed in order to recover correctly from the psychosis I had gone through, which brings me to my next point.

During these years, from eighteen to twenty-two, you usually want to—or in some cases *have to*—go to school. I had dropped out of school by this point, but I wanted to pick up correspondence and finish school that way. I'll admit that school can get pretty strenuous no matter who you are. For me, at the time, it would take me a whole year just to get 2.5 credits. That should have taken me a half year normally. And I was putting in long hours every day. It was just hard to work on the schoolwork through the confusion, irritability, and tiredness I constantly felt. Thank goodness I didn't have to work on top of that also. All that stress would have crushed me. This is another reason I am grateful for the disability checks I received.

# SATAN VERSUS GOD

I don't care if people say you're using your bipolar disorder as an excuse. "Shut up!" is what I want to say and have said to these people. Seriously, you don't say to a dying cancer patient who is having trouble walking, "Get it yourself. Stop using cancer as an excuse that you can't get up yourself," after they asked you for the remote control. I'm serious. It's the same thing if a person is mentally ill.

I was having trouble looking a *unique young lady* in the eyes once. She asked me why I could never look her in the eyes, so I gave her my true, honest, best explanation. I told her earlier in the conversation that I had bipolar disorder, so to bring bipolar disorder up at this time wasn't out of the ordinary. I told her, "Well, probably from my bipolar disorder, I have depression. I am experiencing that right now, and a symptom of depression is loss of eye contact." The explanation seemed simple enough to me. "Don't use that as an excuse," she said. I told her, "It's not an excuse. It's just a fact."

Then I thought, *Come up with a cure for depression and then tell me not to use it as an excuse because then there will be a reason I shouldn't be experiencing what I am.*

An excuse is only an excuse when something can be done and you're not doing it, and you're usually not doing it out of laziness.

It's a mental illness, people. Just because you can't understand it, it doesn't mean it's not a problem. It needs to be taken care of. That's why so many people don't believe in God—because they don't believe it until they see it.

Usually, when doctors or scientists can see something and give an answer to it, people will believe it. That's why cancer is accepted—hated but accepted. That's why mental illness, in a lot of cases, is harder to accept. Brain scans can't pick it up. The only way you know it exists is because a lot of people started experiencing many of the same symptoms and they called it something. At first, they called it manic depression. Now it's bipolar disorder. Mental illnesses are scary because doctors don't know how to deal with them and they are hard to explain.

I just think it's Satan at work. While I believe God allows bad things to happen to people for good reasons, that thought also leaves it open for me to believe that all bad things come from Satan. I often wonder if back in Bible times, when they talked about demon-possessed people scratching themselves with rocks and letting out loud yells, full of rage so the whole city could hear them, with extra strength to take on seven men at once, these people were just what we now call bipolar—a little tamed down, of course, now, although maybe not tamed down in all cases. I have heard stories of men who have bipolar disorder and it took seven policemen to take that one bipolar patient out. I also have let out some pretty rage-filled yells before.

The pictures I get from the Bible seem a bit more intense, though, and they're called demons. Have we just named it bipolar disorder now? I still believe fully that God can completely remove bipolar disorder from your life, whether it's over a period of time or instantly, that he definitely has given us a miracle in itself, and that's modern medicine. Medicine doesn't always work, but it certainly will try to.

I have a confession to make. I have said hurtful things to people and say hurtful comments, which I hate doing. Afterward, I feel very bad for what I have done. That's exactly, in my eyes, what Satan wants. He wants us to hate on each other, and he wants to tear each other down and feel shame. For me, this is just a challenge I must end by winning. I must overcome this chemical imbalance in my brain that causes me to be destructive, to cause that destruction that Satan longs for. Instead, stand up, and still be kind, gentle, and loving through it all. It's a task I know can be done. Soon, Satan will be gone completely from me, and I will find peace. And I will give it all to God. He is my strength and helps me do all I can do.

Call it what you want—bipolar disorder or demons. They both have one thing in common: they bring upon evil, things that are not positive, things that you don't like. God does not want us to worry, to be anxious or apathetic. God wants us to be the opposite of all of those. While we're up against these things, let's learn from them with all our might. Let's fight the battle. Take everything that Bipolar Is giving you and filter it through a grinder. Make it into what it hates. It wants to be mean. Be nice. It wants you to be anxious. Breathe deep. It wants you to have angry outbursts. Hug gentle.

Put to death Satan's schemes. You're a machine at work, with self-conflict. If we all fought our own battles and helped each other, we wouldn't be fighting against each other at all. If you're mad at something and want to attack it, you're probably mad at something you should have been doing first. I'll explain this.

Sometimes, the reasons you get mad at a person are so stupid. For example, a guest walks in the room and you start feeling insecure and you don't get up and say hi. Instead, you let someone else in the party say hi to them. Your heart tells you be kind, but your insecurity tells you no. And you begin thinking harsh thoughts toward the person who acted confidently in approaching the guest in the room, which you wished you had done. The person who approached the guest is now making you mad, but you haven't quite figured out why you are upset; then, later on in the night, you make cheap stabs with hurtful words to knock the person who did approach the guest because you don't know how to deal with your own insecurity. Maybe something evil, something negative, something you don't like is making you want to knock them down to your level. Maybe you wish people understood your pain. If they don't, you will inflict some on them. Maybe the problem is within you. Maybe if you would have gotten up and answered the door and did what you felt you needed to, you wouldn't feel angry against the person who approached the guest. Maybe if you encouraged them in the good they did, their strength could be a temporary crutch for you. Maybe if we could forgive, there would be no need for attack—even if they didn't do anything wrong but you feel they wronged you. We need to put things in a positive and true perspective.

Freedom and stability is ours. Take it and love it. That's the least you could do for those dying kids in Africa and other third-world counties. Be thankful for what you have. Give. Yes, keep giving and don't stop. I can't relate to kids in third-world countries as much as I would like to. I live in a country with so much material it makes it hard. I would like to give a message to those of you with a lot of money. It's not always about your giving. What you can do for those kids in third-world countries is just simply be thankful for what you have. If you, with so much money, are 100 percent thankful for what you have, I would feel a whole lot more comforted. (Not to say you guys don't already.) I wouldn't even expect you guys to give, but if you did, I would feel love and forever feel gratitude toward the person who gave it me to if I were a third-world orphan. If I was given something, I would accept it with loving hands. That's part of being loving—giving someone a chance to give a gift. Accept gifts with gracious, loving hands.

At almost every student/teacher get-together there has been at my school this year, Mrs. W, one of the professors, has sent me home with arms full of food. This loving gift was greatly appreciated, and this was food that I already had at home. Yes, being a college student, this did help out a lot, but her loving gift always made me a bit happier. A lot of the time, what makes up happy is not the actual gift but the thought.

When I had no means to a car or even money for a car, my mom was able to get me one. To make the situation even better, I was given the car during my first year of having my license. I felt even more loved, and that gift will never leave my head. It is of such great value to me.

If a poor, dying kid gets $200, some food, an education, a key to the gate out of poverty, there is not a doubt in my mind that if this kid has a heart, and even if he doesn't, he will never forget what some stranger did for him.

I have been in only one fistfight my whole life. That was in grade nine. He was making fun of me constantly every day, or at least every time I saw him. The thing he would use to make fun of me was the comment, "Taff's a goof!" or some comment like that. He finally said it again, except all his big friends were there. I felt that this time, if they saw him making fun of me and I did not retaliate, they would join and start in on the rip fest and then eventually they would gang up on me physically. So I ran at him, pushed him, and told him to shut up. All his friends ordered a fight to take place behind the store down the road. So there we were. He whooped me. I had my first black eye. This was before bipolar disorder, and I still acted in anger. Am I Jesus? No! I can try to be though! I was wrong for fighting.

Fear and pride drove my actions—two things I only need a little of. You see, I need pride in my Jesus and fear of my God. If I had this attitude, then maybe things would be different. Instead, we delivered pointless blows to each other's head. Thank God I wasn't the president of my country that was bombed because, with fear and pride trying to attack me, I don't know what I would do. I would have the fear of, *If you don't attack, you will be attacked again. Then, if that happens, all of your own people will turn on you.* Then my pride would say, *They took down something special to me and my country. They can't do that.* Doing the right thing would be almost impossible. God be with whomever is the leader of their country. If you become proud of Christ, you will be confident in Christ and hopefully reach a point where you aren't afraid to die for what you believe. Do you give up? No! Fight the battle inside, and make peace outside. While us citizens and people with bipolar disorder fight to live, people are fighting against each other. Wait! Even in Iraq, there are people like me who have bipolar disorder. Hmm. Then I pray for this situation. When things seem out of control, all I can do is pray.

# CLIFFORD WHIITING BEERS AND WHY AMERICANS SHOULD BE PROUD OF HIM

There is hope for suicide rates to decrease. We all know there is. We have to. If we don't hope, we need to start.

Let me share a story about our friend Clifford Whiiting Beers. During his suicidal low, Clifford tried to commit suicide. Here's how he tried, and here's how he survived, and here's what he lived to conclude about the experience. The story starts with Clifford on the fourth story of his mother's house.

> Shortly after noon, dinner having been served, my mother entered the room and asked me if she should bring me some dessert. I assented. It was not that I cared for the dessert; I had no appetite. I wished to get her out of the room, for I believed myself to be on the verge of another attack. She left at once. I knew that in two or three minutes

she would return. The crisis seemed at hand. It was now or never for liberation. She had probably descended one of three flights of stairs when, with the mad desire to dash my brains out on the pavement below, I rushed to that window which was directly over the flag walk. Providence must have guided my movements, for in some otherwise unaccountable way, on the very point of hurling myself out bodily, I chose to drop feet foremost instead. With my fingers I clung for a moment to the sill. Then I let go. In falling my body turned so as to bring my right side toward the building. I struck the ground a little more than two feet from the foundation of the house, and at least three to the left of the point from which I started. Missing the stone pavement by not more than three or four inches, I struck on comparatively soft earth. My position must have been almost upright, for both heels struck the ground squarely. The concussion slightly crushed one heel bone and broke most of the small bones in the arch of each foot, but there was no mutilation of the flesh. As my feet struck the ground my right hand struck hard against the front of the house, and it is probable that these three points of contact, dividing the force of the shock, prevented my back from being broken. As it was, it narrowly escaped a fracture and, for several weeks afterward, it felt as if powdered glass had been substituted for cartilage between the vertebrae.[17]

His conclusion to it all was that "many a suicide might be averted if the person contemplating it could find the proper assistance when such a crisis impends,"

Clifford went on from his experiences to found a foundation that is now called Mental Health America, which is a program to help the mentally ill live better lives. Clifford underwent poor treatment in pychiatrict hospitals, which motivated him to start a program as the one he started. He founded this movement in 1909. His movement was revolutionary at his time.

# HOW YOU CAN HELP A PERSON IN DISTRESS

Never let a loner be a loner. You don't know what he is thinking while he stares at the tall building. It may not be about the architecture. He may be considering jumping off the tall building. Show love and say hi.

Listening is key. Prayer is important. When things are out of your hands, you can only give it to a bigger power. But be alert. You may need to take action, but listening is key. They just want to talk. Always show them more love then more than ever. Shower them with encouragement, and don't stop. Hugs, kisses, presents, and thoughtful comments will all save a person from the brink. Be compassionate.

# SHORT FILM

This chapter will tie into the idea I had earlier about bipolar disorder being a demon. The idea has been mention by people before me. I'm just deeply considering it as a possibility and will lay out a scenario I refer to as short film that should bring the idea to life that Bipolar is a demon. Whatever your opinion is, what I do know for sure is that what both demons and bipolar disorder have in common is they are bad, to put it lightly. Both are not from God.

Based on the scripture of Acts 19:11–20:

> God did extraordinary miracles through Paul so that even handkerchiefs and aprons that had touched him were taken to the sick and their illnesses were cured and the evil spirits left them.
>
> Some Jews who went around driving out evil spirits tried to invoke the name of the Lord Jesus over those who were demon-possessed. They would say, "In the name of Jesus, whom Paul

preaches, I command you to come out." Seven sons of Sceva, a Jewish chief priest, were doing this. (One day) the evil spirit answered them, "Jesus I know, and I know about Paul, but who are you?" Then the man who had the evil spirit jumped on them and overpowered them all. He gave them such a beating that they ran out of the house naked and bleeding.

When this became known to the Jews and Greeks living in Ephesus, they were all seized with fear and the name of the Lord Jesus was held in high honor. Many of those who believed now came and openly confessed their evil deeds. A number who had practiced sorcery brought their scrolls together and burned them publicly. When they calculated the value of the scrolls, the total came to fifty thousand drachmas. In this way the Word of the Lord spread widely and grew in power.

## My Summary of Acts 19:11–20

A man who is demon possessed jumps a priest and his seven sons. Because of this, a whole town begins to turn to Jesus and honor his name in fear of God. Even people who practiced witchcraft threw out their scrolls.

## The Idea of the Film

The idea I want to aim at is more of the subplot of the story: Who was this demon-possessed man? What kind of life did this demon-possessed man live before this event took place?

What if he was what we know now as a bipolar person experiencing one of the *highest* states of mania?

What if, before his giant manic episode and psychosis, he lived a quiet life all alone in the mountains? There, in the mountains, he had periods of normalness and periods of hyper mania.

This man's thoughts could have been learned about because he kept a journal. When his demon or bipolar disorder was bearable, he would write and describe the feelings he had, that he was being led to do something for God. He just didn't know what. He was scared. We refer to his problem as a demon, like it was referred to in the Bible, but maybe over time the same symptoms demon-possessed people had in the Bible—cutting themselves with rocks (Mark 5:5), social problems (Matt. 9:32), loud yelling (Luke 4:32–34, 8:26–28), loss of self-worth (Luke 8:26–28), feeling out of control (Luke 9:41–43), attacking people (Matthew 8:28, Acts 19 11:19), and keeping yourself in solitude (Luke 8:28–30)—were all things that some doctor called manic depression after a while and then later, because of the stigma manic depression carried, soon, the name changed to bipolar disorder.

These people were ordinary people just like us, suffering and some experiencing more extreme symptoms than others. But that is how it is for people with bipolar disorder or for anybody who has anything wrong with them. Doesn't there always seem to be someone better or more worse off than you? Just a side note: Jesus healed these people (Matthew 4:23–25, 8:16, 8:30–32).

As we continue the plot of the short film,the demon-possessed man, between his thoughts and journal writings he wrote, he often cut himself with rocks, mutilated animals, and let out scary yells. But behind all this was a gentleman who knew and loved the Lord. How he discovered the Lord was once while he crept around the city, watching what was going on, hoping not to be spotted, in fear of humiliation. He had seen a man name Paul, who spoke all about Jesus. This is when our main character (the demon-possessed man) latched on to Jesus.

Before this man became demonized, or induced with bipolar disorder, and even knew about Jesus he studied the Torah. A replay of the day this strange activity occurred will be shown at this point.

This day the Lord had planned for him, was coming closer. He knew it. He felt it. So, as he felt directed, he walked into town and there was Sceve and his seven sons, healing in Jesus' name when they, in their minds, didn't believe Jesus even existed. When they tried to heal; the demon possessed man (our main character) what he did, he did not want to do, but while he did it, he did not even realize he was doing so. That's when he severely beat Sceva and his seven sons.

After this event, our main character found himself on the edge of a cliff, curled up in a ball. He looked more at peace than he ever has. This leaves the audience with the idea that he has now been healed. The town never sees or hears of this man again.

The idea of this film is to prove that God uses bad circumstances and turns them into good ones. It's to ask the question, Why does God let good people suffer? And to help us think and hopefully feel compassion for these people in the Bible who were demon possessed.

This is an entirely fictional story, besides the Acts 19:11–20 premises.

The movie will end showing many coming to Christ, and that's is the non-fiction part of the story.

# ARE YOU OVERSENSITIVE? OVERSENSITIVITY LEADS TO NEGATIVITY

I am going to have to answer yes. At times, I can be. Please allow me to share a few stories that have given me positive evidence that yes, indeed, I have been oversensitive at times. I can also share a few stories that make me seem not so oversensitive. But for now, we will stick to the stories that prove I have been oversensitive. Embrace yourselves. You're in for a treat. Newspapers, talk shows, and soap operas are so popular, and they are so full of negative information at times. We like to hear negative things at times, some of us more than others, right? Don't get down on yourselves. You're not a sadist quite yet. Hearing the negative allows you to learn that there is a positive side to things. This why I will show you a few negative sides to myself, involving times I have been oversensitive.

Hopefully, through me sharing a weakness, you can learn from it or gain courage from my weakness. The same works if anyone shares their weaknesses. By someone sharing a weakness, it is for the listener to realize that maybe he or she has something in common with the person sharing or for the listener to self-discover his own weakness because to better yourself, you have to admit what's wrong first, which we all already know, of course. Now let's just do it.

I remember a recent, specific incident. I was getting off the C train, and before the doors had opened, I noticed two people standing outside the doors, waiting to get in. So I thought, *Okay, I'll get out of the C train, say a friendly hi; walk by; and it will be a very nice, friendly moment and very simple too.* This was a big step for me at the time, trying to be more social.

Then, just as the doors opened, the one lady looked at me and moved way over to the side, not giving me a chance to say hi the way I had planned it. This deeply hurt my feelings. I felt angry. I could not communicate to her what I wanted to say. I felt like I was in the way because she had to move—which I wasn't. She didn't have to move, but that's beside the point. Most of all, I felt I had bad communication skills and that my brain was too slow to react to her moving. I wish my brain had accepted that she had moved and had still been able to say hi. Anyways, yes, I know this seems like a very small ordeal, but little things like that just always happen to me and leave me feeling irritable. It's something I have to put up/deal with. I especially have to deal with them because I know they can be dealt with and will not/cannot remain forever.

One thought I have came up with is that I get hurt when people misunderstand me. For example, I'm at a banquet that is beautifully decorated and I'm sitting down with six others and it's just a beautiful time. The conversation carries on, and I ask my professor how our class did on an assignment that the class had just handed in. (I will admit that when I asked him, I was feeling frustrated for a reason I did not know. This usually leads to a higher chance for your feelings to be hurt because you're not happy.) The conversation carried on, and he said "*You* did great!" Well, I hadn't asked him how *I* did. I asked him how we did. I felt as if his comment was made because he thought I wanted some forced encouragement from him, which I didn't. I just wanted to seriously know how the whole class did. But I panicked. I felt under pressure. Everyone was listening, and I felt ridiculed in front of everyone. *How dare he brush me off like that? That's not what I meant!* I thought to myself. Sometimes it is okay to feel that way, but it's better if you can communicate how you feel. So, after reflecting on this situation after dinner, I thought, well, I should have just said, "Oh did I?" (nicely) and then said, "That's great, but how did everybody else do?" This would let him know that

I seriously wanted to know how everyone did, not just me.

Instead, the conversation went like this. I said, "I know I did great." Then I must have been silent for a second because he had time to reply before I could say what I wanted to, which, now reflecting, I think, *Wow! Maybe I was being a slow thinker,* another negative thought that I'm sure added to the already negative thinking cycle. (The negative thoughts don't stop coming, eh? Seems like you have to always fight them off.) He replied with some constructive criticism, which, if you know anything about oversensitivity, even simple constructive criticism, especially in front of people, is hard for you.

He replied, "You need to let other people compliment you. Don't do it yourself!" Okay. Yes, this is a valid point. Thank you. It was a great comment. It really was. But in my head, I was choked because this had gotten way of track of what I was trying to say.

So now I argued, "I'm not complimenting myself. I just said I know I did well. That is just self-confidence, like if someone asked you how you did on something and you said great, right? If you think you did do great, right?" Then he said, "Yes. You're arguing back…"

So now this turned into an almost heated argument. Being stubborn, I finally said—and by this time I don't even know what I was thinking but eventually I did get out what I was trying to say; it just took awhile—"No. You messed up first by not answering my question. I asked how the whole class did. Not just me. I don't even want this to be about me."

Note: By pointing out others, you risk the chance of offending someone. He, being the loving person he is, didn't take offence, which I'm thankful for, and answered "Oh. Well, they all did good." I finally got the answer I was looking for and, in the meantime, learned how—if not aware of your oversensitivity in a situation—not communicating properly can lead to confusion, which can lead to hurtful words being said. This is why I hate Satan.

If you really care or not, if you are oversensitive or not, take the *Are You Oversensitive Test.*

### The Are You Oversensitive Test

- When remarks are made about your personality, do you feel offended?
- Is criticism very hard to handle?
- Does loud noise or loud music make you feel badly irritated or angry?
- Do you feel other people's pain and suffering a lot more then the average person?
- Do you have a smaller body size than your peers? (Smaller body types are, 99 percent of the time, very sensitive.)

- Do you stop for more than three minutes to observe an accident anywhere in order to watch?
- Are high or low temperatures almost intolerable to you?
- Does it take a lot of working out/exercise to gain muscle mass?
- Do little things send you into mood swings?

If you answer yes to most of those questions, pray about it. And also, don't get too discouraged because feeling other people's pain can also be called empathy, and that's a great gift. A great friend of empathy is compassion. Basically, compassion often needs empathy. For example, you feel for someone or something. This is empathy. And if you act on it by trying to make the situation better, that is compassion.

Jesus always was doing this. There's a story of him and his apostles. His disciples had just came back from teaching the good news about Jesus, and they were telling Jesus all about it. Because people had been coming and going all day to see Jesus, he and his disciples hadn't had a chance to eat, and to solve that, the disciples and him went to go to a solitary place for rest (Mark 6:30–31).

Jesus and the crew took the boat and headed for their quiet place. The crowd noticed this and beat them there by foot. Jesus looked at the crowd and had compassion for them because they were like sheep without a shepherd. So he began teaching them many things. By this time, it was late in the day, so his disciples came to him.

> "This is a remote place," they said, "and it's already very late. Send the people away so they can go to the surrounding countryside and villages and buy themselves something to eat." But he answered, "You give them something to eat."
>
> Mark 6:35–36

They said to him,"Are you nuts?" Well, not quite. They were more specific with their comment.

> "That would take eight months of a man's wages! Are we to go and spend that much on bread and give it to them to eat?" "How many loaves do you have?" he asked. "Go and see." When they found out, they said, "Five—and two fish."
>
> Then Jesus directed them to have all the people sit down in groups on the green grass. So they sat down in groups of hundreds and fifties. Taking the five loaves and the two fish and looking up to heaven, he gave thanks and broke the loaves. Then he gave them to his disciples to set before the people. He also divided the two fish among them all. They all ate and were satisfied, and the disciples picked up twelve basketfuls of broken

> pieces of bread and fish. The number of the men who had eaten was five thousand.
>
> Mark 6:35–43

What I'm trying to say is having empathy can be great. Being sensitive to someone *can* be great.

At that same banquet I was at, a single mother, who I have seen around school all year working her but off, got rewarded the women's half of a scholarship award, and I knew this lady worked so hard all year, trying to raise a child on her own, battling through personal struggles, and hammering away while, at the same time, carrying a full time college course load.

When she got called up, tears came to my eyes. I was so proud at what she had accomplished, and I knew she was feeling the same thing. It was a privilege to congratulate her on her award.

Those feeling you get, the ones you share with others, those oversensitive feelings, they may be called, are sometimes used for good things like feeling the emotions of someone who has just accomplished something great. Being oversensitive is not just a negative thing. It can be when slight criticism feels like a hammer to the head, but it can be good when it comes to positive emotions.

I would say that most people share similar feelings at some point in their life, but some are just more sensitive than others. Some it takes a lot to feel anything.

Others can't wake up without feeling extreme emotions. It's important to deal with the negative emotions we get, the ones you know are senseless, because after the occurrence, you look back and feel ashamed and put your head in your hands and scream and then come up for air with a bright red face. How can you be sensible while feeling like a fool? How can you feel sensible while all your emotions are pulling you to do what is wrong, especially when the decision has to be made quickly? If you carefully think and spend time alone in prayer or meditation, you can set firm morals for yourself that will help you discern what is wrong and what is right, even when you're feeling the worst emotions. You need to get alone and be on your own and talk it over with God. Just say everything on your heart to him, every problem you have, and then ground a lot of your thought in the biblical truth, which is God's Word, and you will set morals in you that will satisfy your soul. When you're with people, it's harder to do that because you're distracted by what is around you. What is around you might be influential. Because of this, you will act more instinctively or act by what feels good. It's not until you get alone and feel the pain you're feeling that you haven't been noticing all day that you will find the truth with what is going on inside of you and the truth about what is right and wrong. Once you have brought yourself to a quiet place where you will feel the pain, a place that isn't full of bright lights, rides, entertainment, things that will numb you to your pain, you can find truth. Sure, have fun doing all the things listed above, but do them after you get alone time. Be brave. Try to sit alone. Feel the loneliness burn if that is what you're hiding. Then pour it out to God. It is then that you will fight your thoughts, and determine what is wrong and right! And it is then when you will be equipped to go out in the world to have some fun and come across a situation in the heat of the moment and say, "Nuh-uh-uh. I ain't doing that." It will be the time you spend alone that will build your strength, the strength that will allow you to be around people and stand up for what you believe in. Extravert or introvert, we all need time to assess. We all need time to hear God.

## ESCAPISM

I noticed that, since bipolar disorder has really shown itself in my life, I have been looking for escape. My escape at first was drugs and girls and then clubs. Now I'm off drugs and staying away from my old ways of escape. Even TV was an escape once I got off the drugs, and now I don't even watch that much TV. But, still, I find myself looking for escape. My mind seems to have been renewed so much in Christ, so I never find a bad escape that my morals will allow me to go through, which is a good thing.

But I was at a family gathering today, and I was having a good time. I truly was. But I found myself walking around the house, looking for an escape. Then I finally said to myself, *Jason, this is your life. This is how you feel right now. You have to live it.* And sure enough, moments came in my day where my mind came off the pain, like when I sat at the table and had an intense conversation with my granddad and a friend of the family named Jason. I think we were talking about computers. But our brains were really clicking, and we were just firing back information back and forth at each other as fast as a ping pong ball in the world championships.

This gave me enough *release* I'll call it for now, to make it through the rest of the night. So, stick with it! Finding release from your pain is there for you. It's waiting around the corner for you if you keep on pushing in the right direction.

## LEARNING TO LOVE THE PAIN

Take delight in your sufferings, Christ will not let your suffering go in vain. Learn to enjoy the pain you go through because you know that your suffering is going to make you stronger. This does not mean afflicting pain on yourself. This is not right. Getting stronger through pain is even shown when a person gets stitches. He goes through pain to get better. I think bipolar disorder can be a lot like that. You go through immense pain, but in the end, you're stronger, you're wiser, you may have more knowledge, you're more disciplined, and the list goes on and on.

# DISCIPLINE

If you're experiencing feelings of absolute dragon fire breathed anger and you learn to not react negatively to that, you begin to discipline yourself. Now, I understand when you're at the point in your life when bipolar disorder seems to be really acting up and acting positively with your anger seems to be impossible. I'll assure you it isn't impossible, but it is really hard. I wasn't able to do it at first, so, good luck with that. May God be with you.

But there are many ways to release that anger in a positive way. Sometimes, that way doesn't always work. Like, for example, I will feel really angry and, depending on the circumstance, I might choose to read the Bible. The words from the page instantly ease my tension, and it doesn't fix the problem completely, but it relaxes me real quickly, and at the same time, I was learning.

Usually, I find the Bible best to read in those situations specially because it's full of such intense lines and stories and it's more effective to ease me. There are other times when just anything helped, even the newspaper.

Then there have been times when I have gotten frustrated and acted out negatively, and halfway through my frustration, I caught myself and *did* contain it.

For example, I played for the Rocky Mountain Rams college basketball team. In my first year of school, this was a great privilege. In this particular game, the half was reaching toward its end. I was on the court for not too long, and coached pulled me off. This set off the anger. Now, remember, normally, that won't make you to mad unless you're Michael Jordan and it's overtime. But when you're battling all your emotions and playing a bad game, things like that just set you off. Because, at the time, I was trying really hard to play a good game of basketball. I do have the ability to play incredibly and really benefit the team, but, this game, I couldn't seem to focus. Nothing was going my way. I was beginning to get really mad at myself, which is where most of my anger comes from. Let me rearticulate this. My anger comes from *me* being mad at myself. A lot of the time, I'm starting to find that's where most people's anger comes from—they are mad at themselves for something—but not in all cases.

So now that you're updated on how I felt about my anger, let's rewind a little. Let's back it up to the second quarter, just before coach pulled me off. So it's second quarter, and I'm already battling with my mind, trying to get my mind focused to play better. I started to feel like it was finally coming. I had some energy. I felt alert. Then coach pulls me off. *Darn!* I said in my mind. I sat on the bench and kept thinking about how mad I was. I kept allowing my mind to dwell on what just happened over and over again, making me even madder and madder.

Thank goodness Coach can't read minds or I would have stayed right where I was sitting, on the dreaded, cold, fearful bench that I was supposed to be warming up. Because the coach, at this point in his life, wasn't reading minds (I hope not anyways), he put me back on. My shining, glorious moment, I'm so full of energy, which is a good thing, and I'm ready to put that ball in the net. The kind of energy I had at the time, seeing how I was just angry was a temperamental type of energy that could have been used to fuel my anger or fuel the life in me. If I chose to fuel the life in me the repercussion is huge, it could lead to the contagious spread of joy.

There I am, the stands full, the lights brightening up the whole gym, my shoes are tied tight, and you will never guess it. The ref makes a bad call on me. I know you're probably thinking, *You're just saying that because every athlete says the ref made a bad call at least once in their lives.* To be honest, I still don't even know what I was called for. Then a teammate grabbed me and said, "Settle down." I pushed his arm off—which I should have never done, especially in front of everyone—and then the coach pulled me off. I got in his face. He pointed to the bench and said sternly, "Sit down!" Although I really didn't want to and I wanted to keep yelling at him, I obeyed his orders and sat down. I began to think a bit better. How could I make myself less angry, and help the team? So I picked up a ball and began to dribble it. Normally, you can do that when you on the bench, but the gym I was in was small, so the coach said stop. So I decided to leave the gym and go for a walk. A teammate followed me. He talked to me, and I didn't reply because everything I had to say was not anything that was going to encourage him. Then he finally asked, "What can I do to help you out, man?" He was very compassionate. I didn't know what he could do for me. There wasn't much because I was fighting a spiritual and emotional battle here, so I just said, "Let's pray." He did. He laid out some nice lines to my Lord. And then I said, "Thank you." *Buzz!* It was halftime.

I went for a walk during halftime, and I guess while the team was having a meeting in the changing room the coached asked where I was. The teammates stood up for me, and I'm pretty sure they sympathetically said I was going for a walk. The only reason I believe they stood up for me was because the coach's next words were, "Jason's starting next half." I could not see the coach starting me next half unless he looked around at some of my teammates and saw some forgiving eyes. Something inside of him chose to take a risk by putting me back on the court. I came back to find that out, thinking, *Man, now I really can't screw up. He's showing me such grace.*

I got out on the court. I focused all that energy, which was very temperamental at the time. I was still not too worried because I felt a lot of discipline at that moment. I was not going to let anyone down. Thank the Lord I got two steals and two baskets in two minutes. The fans were roaring, and then I went downhill from there, in term of points, but at least I tried to set a good example. I thank my team for being a great bunch of guys. They were awesome, making me laugh a lot throughout the year, and a bunch of other crazy things happened that made things memorable for me. Thanks, guys! All of you, each and every one of you, made a difference in my life somehow. Thanks, men.

# REJECTION

The feeling of rejection is hard to deal with. Today, I went to go re-obtain my position at Camped I used to work at, and I was denied. Do I feel that bipolar disorder got in the way of this? A little bit. The rejection killed me, although I did hate the job. I didn't really want to work there anyways, but I still tried really hard to do the best job I could, but my best wasn't good enough for them.

I didn't think if I was rejected I would feel so much anxiety, but I did. When I got home, I tried e-mailing a friend and my chest got heavy and I found it hard to breathe. So I went and prayed and then fell asleep for three hours. I usually don't sleep away my pains, but whatever. I didn't have much sleep last night, so, in a way, I was making up for lost sleep.

Nonetheless, sleep was only an escape from reality. While you're sleeping, you don't have to feel your pain. You see, when I woke up from that sleep, I didn't feel much even then, but as soon as I got out of bed, it all came running back. *The anxiety isn't as bad right now, but my heart aches incredibly.* Those were my thoughts when I woke up. I think we take loss harder than we think we take it. I was quick to shrug off my loss and say it was no big deal to my friends, but, *Is this yet another rejection done to me?* I thought.

It's worse getting rejected when you actually try. If you don't try, it hurts as well, but you also feel guilty for not trying, less than feeling flat-out rejected. If you tried your hardest, what is there to do? Well, for me, I am just going to keep on walking, and I am not going to stop!

The lousy part about it all is it seems like I just started getting better and my bipolar disorder symptoms started going away. Definite improvement was seen from last year to this year. Seeing my employers and some of the people I worked with last year this year reminded me people always aren't accepting. Last year, I was so lost I didn't notice, but this year, it just clicked. *Wow! I really don't want to be here.*

I always had a strong character. It caused a lot of trouble for me in school growing up. When I got bipolar disorder and became depressed, I became very quiet and didn't say much because my brain was going through heavy duty changes. Now I'm starting to speak up a bit, be my outgoing self a bit more; but just like in school, they want to shut me up. Maybe authority doesn't like to hear opinion. The right kind of authority does. The best kind of authority does listen. Will you rise to the occasion, schoolteachers?

After going through some of what bipolar disorder had me go through, it opened my eyes to realize why God must be so mad. We (humans) *don't* get along good enough. You know what I'm saying? There's always somebody trying to stir something up. The doctors tell me one of my symptoms is confusion. I'm beginning to realize that, hey, I'm not the only one swept up with mass confusion. It seems like the whole world is.

For example, here it is. If I do something and in my heart I meant it to be pure and just, another person may interpret that as an insult. Then they deal with that insult in an aggressive manner. This is confusion.

How do you react to a mentally ill person? How do you handle an outrageous scene? To go on further with this question, I'm going to have to go back to shortly after I was diagnosed with bipolar disorder. I joined a mental illness support group. There were about seven of us who got together and did activities, such as going to the YMCA. On this joyous day of going to the YMCA, one of my friends in the group was going through a psychosis. He has schizophrenia and was seeing colors and objects; he was hallucinating. The rest of us were in the deep end of the pool, playing catch with the football. It was while playing catch I caught my eye on Dianna, the organizer, in the shallow end, tucked in the corner, looking down into the pool at my friend. I thought maybe he didn't feel comfortable hanging out with us, that maybe felt a bit of an outsider, so I thought I would invite him to come with us and maybe this would help. As I got closer, I realized his eyes were in the back of his head. He was hallucinating big time. The sky was red to him, he told us. His senses were clearly all disorientated. Dianna asked me to bring him to the changing room to get changed, so I took one of the other guys, and we escorted him in. He was able to get changed, and he was doing an excellent job, but I think the voices got louder right about the time he took off his bathing suit, because right there he looked to the sky and kind of rubbed his eyes while shouting things. He wasn't shouting too loud, but he was defiantly in pain and naked. What blew me away was how everyone knew this guy was in some type of trouble but just stood there and stared at him and gave him extremely weird looks.

He could still hear me, so I just took his arm and guided him toward his clothes and walked him through with my words how to get dressed because he was battling something quite large in his head at the moment.

What ticks me off is people get so confused. They think, *Uh oh. He's going to do something so crazy,* and they don't know how to react. The truth is, this guy was the gentlest guy I have probably ever met, and he was not even close to hurting people. He was just hearing things in his head and seeing things. He still was conscious, he could still hear, and he just needed help. If he wasn't with us and was off on his own, I would be scared for the wellbeing of that brave man, but he loves to bike and he's still human.

I am where I am, and you must deal with me where I am, not where I should be. I have worked hard to get where I'm at today, and if they don't want me working with them, there's nothing I can do about it. I would be a good asset to the team. I would do a good job. I work hard, and I constantly try to improve on myself.

Some people are born confident, some people are born confident and then lose it all one day, and others are born with no confidence and must always work hard.

Confidence, as a character attribute, is great. You may lose it one day. Having no confidence isn't so great, but you can gain it all back. If you make a decision and stick to it, this will create confidence. If you work hard enough to satisfy your own heart, leaving yourself self-assured, this will create confidence. When you know your limits and you have reached them, you know something. Knowing something makes you confident. Experience can prepare you. Preparation makes you confident. Everyone needs confidence. Reach for it out in the rainbow, past the pot of gold.

# DEALING WITH PEOPLE WHO HAVE BIPOLAR DISORDER

## Random Public

I will start my first point off with the word *compassion*. Compassion is ultimately what you need to use to deal with anyone. Personally, I don't care how you treat me. I'll be content whatever the circumstance. I have been treated at all different levels while here on earth, and it is possible to remain content in all of them. You can learn to be content whatever the circumstance (Philippians 4:11). Paul, a man who went through many trials, also shares his thoughts on contentment.

> I know what it is to be in need, and I know what it is to have plenty. I have learned the secret of being content in any and every situation, whether well fed or hungry, whether living in plenty or in want. I can do anything through him who gives me strength.
>
> Philippians 4:12–13

Where my anger comes from is the way I see other people with bipolar disorder being treated. I see it all the time. It's just not good. I don't know if people mean to do it or not, but have you ever been sitting in a public area, maybe a library or someplace, and you may be reading or just waiting your turn in line, and you overhear the lady behind the desk wherever you maybe, helping the oncoming people coming her way. Then, every once in a while, you hear her, and she starts talking really loud and very slow and tries extra hard to make her words as clear as possible? You think as you're reading your book or looking the other direction, *Oh. She must be dealing with a kid.* Then you look over and it's a full-grown adult.

If you're bipolar, scared, quiet, and depressed and a lady starts yelling at you like that, you get kind of freaked out. The depression might be so low you can't defend yourself, and you just softly answer back, at the same time feeling a bit put down by the way you're being talked to. If this has happened to you and you were a perfectly strong adult at the time, you just replied back to her very sternly so she knew who she was dealing with.

Yesterday, I was at the fair. Like an angel, an older lady who looked half homeless and was missing all her teeth, came to me and asked for two dollars so she could buy a coffee. I was at a fair. I had already spent a lot of money and was down on myself for that, so

I said, "No. Sorry. I spent it all at the fair." She said, "Nice teeth." I say she was like angel because, at that exact moment, I left all my friends from the fair to be alone because I was feeling very low, and she just came to talk to me at that time, plus her telling me I had nice teeth made me feel a lot better. My conscience caught up to me. I couldn't believe I had spent all that money on stupid rides and games when I could have given it to the poor and now, when one of them is asking me for just a drink, I have to say no. *No way. I have to give if God's investment plan is as good as he says it is, then why not?.*

"Give, and it will be given to you. A good measure, pressed down, shaken together and running over, will be poured into your lap. For with the measure you use, it will be measured to you," (Luke 6:38).

*Then I'm not really losing out on anything,* I thought. Plus, she needed it more than I did. Turns out she didn't know where to get coffee at the fair, and I happened to remember. It was a small place tucked away. I don't blame her for not knowing where it was. I took her there, and she started preaching *to me.* I thought maybe I could share some biblical truth, but she began teaching me. This was shocking and humbling at the same time. We finally got her drink and we parted ways, and she was at least not thirsty anymore.

I tell you this story because, although I have no proof she was bipolar, it was clear and evident to anyone she had some type of mental illness. My guess was she had untreated bipolar disorder for a very long time, but schizophrenia could be a possibility. That's not important though. What I'm trying to get at is my friend who came up to me after she had left said, "Who was that lady you were with? Man, she's a real kook, eh?"

I said, "Actually, I thought she was a very sweet lady."

"Oh. What did she want?"

"A drink!"

"You give it to her?"

"Yep."

"Why would you do that?"

"I like to give I guess."

"Oh. Cool."

I was not mad at this guy for looking down on this girl. He was young only sixteen. He had a lot to learn. Later, walking home, he had to go the same way, so we talked and I told him how important it is to give and how he needs to learn how to handle people like that. I told him she probably had a mental illness. He hadn't thought of it that way before. She was just a kook to him. I think a little bit of his heart opened up and understood what compassion is and how helping people like that can be fun. You have never heard a better story than the story of a person on the streets—whether it's sad or just funny, they can be educational.

"Mental disorders accounted for 52 percent of acute care hospitalizations among the homeless in 2005-2006." A lot of the homeless are mentally ill. If we treat them with compassion, it will give them a chance to recover. Every time they are ignored and treated poorly, it adds to their problems and makes it more difficult for them to get out of their problems. It's important to understand people because when you do they become less scary.

# SAYING SORRY

One day, as I walked down the street in my sorrows, something clicked in me. Amidst the anxiety, anger, and sorrow I feel throughout the day, when someone says sorry to me, it can soothe it all. The sorry could be for any meaningless thing or little mistake a person made against me. Sometimes, a person says sorry and I wonder if they can actually see my sorrow and they are sorry for that rather then being sorry for something they have actually done.

When someone close to you dies, you are told by friends and even family that they are sorry for your loss. In one incident, I was apologized to with a sorry that came from the sweetest of girls; she soothed my soul with just her voice after she had said sorry. It does soothe me for a quick second, which is enough to enjoy and feel the satisfaction of relief.

Upon pondering this, I thought a few things. One, I thought, *Well, maybe I'm just imagining this,* (which could be true), and the girl who said sorry to me just felt as if she had done wrong and apologized and actually wasn't saying sorry on behalf of my losses. Then I thought, *What a fancy idea that someone would say sorry if they knew you had bipolar disorder or suffered from depression.* How considerate would it be if a bipolar person shared that he or she was bipolar and instead of the reply being "really?" The reply was, "I'm sorry to hear that." How much that would make sense, seeing how the person inflicted went from normal mental function to mentally ill. Seeing how a person had gone through a psychosis which sent him or her from having a grip of reality to losing their grip of reality, the word sorry could mean a lot.

Wouldn't it be appropriate to tell a bipolar or mentally ill person you were sorry to hear of their instability and all the losses that go along with it, their loss of happiness, of normal mental function, of clarity in thought, of peace? All things are attainable to get back, but while a person is experiencing harsh symptoms of bipolar disorder, how easing it would be to hear the words sorry from an understanding, loving person. It is an illness that is hard to understand unless one has it. When someone does not have bipolar disorder, saying sorry would be best approached by empathizing with someone who has bipolar disorder—not feeling sorry for them, but, "Sorry to hear. I wish I could help," as a thought process to go through a civilian's mind who hears of such drama would be best.

Do I find it realistic to say I'm sorry in a situation when one is inflicted with a mental illness? In its place, yes, I'm certainly not insulted if a person is intrigued and does say, "Really?" And no one has ever said they were sorry to me, so I can't say I like to hear that more.

When genuinely apologizing to someone, the effects will be nothing but positive. As said before, when I was apologized to about something that hadn't bothered me in the first place, it still seemed to have brought an easing sense to my chest, which was aching at the time. Looking at what I almost call fact, but realized in some situations, my next statement does not hold true in every situation so I do not call it a fact is the so-called fact, that it is hard to be mad at a sorry person, because they are sorry.

Well, I have said over and over throughout this book that, having bipolar disorder, I have become stronger in many ways of life but would not curse bipolar disorder on anyone. The lonely nights I have spent alone in my turmoil, looking to anything that might cheer me up, whether it's the stars or the moon on a clear night, I would be drowning in unknown sorrows, scared, with my nerves on complete edge while my thoughts raced—no man should have to endure this. I will though, because if a shivering child cold on the street all alone must go through what he goes through, then I will defiantly accept my challenge without complaint. If my challenge is going to make me stronger in the end, I will embrace suffering, especially if, through it, I become stronger, because with that strength, I wish to use it to help someone else who needs it.

I think I'm starting to feel scared of the change that is going on in me. I shouldn't because it's a positive change. But it seems as if I'm coming back to life with a transformed mind, a transformed life, where I feel more relaxed. I'm not sure why I'm scared of the change, but I keep getting glimpses of the improvements throughout the day. Maybe I'm scared because the better I get the more I realize how bad things were for me and how I was acting, and I'm finding it annoying, how I was. Either way, looking back at how much you have improved is a very humbling experience, not shameful at all. I may be scared about how God is going to use me, and his gifts and blessings can almost become overwhelming. God's blessings come usually from obedience to him. After obeying God, Satan may try to overwhelm those who obey God, to make them think they don't deserve his blessing. God thinks whomever he blesses deserves it or he would not bless him otherwise.

Boy, it's tough going through trials, but I'm loving life more because of them. It's tough. I keep learning though that your patient resolution will come. If in a bad situation, if feeling tense, if feeling like people or life circumstances are ganging up on you, if it feels like people are treating you poorly, hey, maybe they are or maybe it's oversensitivity. I find if you're going through pain, be patient, because what goes around seems to come around, but it's not your job to avenge. If people wait patiently during adversity, something positive will happen. Your pain will not happen in vain.

# IRRITABILITY

This stuff creates anger. I hate it, especially when you're *extremely* irritable. I think this is why bipolar people like to isolate themselves, because irritation usually comes from other people. Irritation may start inside the heart, it almost defiantly starts inside the heart, but it seems to feel like it's coming from other people. Other people may bring it out of us. When I was alone, I didn't get irritated too easily, but when people came around, the noise would really irritate me. It was worse at the beginning of my time with bipolar disorder. People who get migraines often describe things this way. They say noises make the headache worse, so maybe people with migraines can relate to this a degree. I'm not sure.

If you can relate to hearing noises that you feel all up the side of your face, and if you can relate to noises that have lost their sweet sound, then you can relate to what I am talking about. An example of that is I even remember times when a running river would annoy me. Not all the time would the running river annoy me though, but there were a few times. If you can relate to hearing every sound there is at the moment you're listening, and they're all only making you mad, then you know what I'm talking about.

It wasn't always the irritability that would drive me nuts. I remember being so sensitive to being close to people that it would throw me for a whirl. For example, as soon as my dad pulled in the driveway after being home alone all morning and afternoon, I felt irritation spread through my body, and it was so tough to go through. I found that talking helped. So if you feel that irritable feeling you get when someone gets close or when you feel their presence near, sometimes talking to the source helps. Like if my dad just came in and walked around and I didn't go talk to him it would get worse. I would get more irritable. But if I went and talked to him, I found that the personal connection helped. Although it seemed scary and felt irritable, like you may blow up on that person, the personal connection helped. Even if getting close to people is hard, you have to go talk to people. You have to put yourself in a community. There's no other way out. There is no escaping your irritation without community. You may be strong, but we all need help. It's true that often, you will find yourself in your best and worst situations when you're in community situations. If trying to be part of a community seems to fail after attempting it the first time, don't fret because one aspect of community is that people will fail in front of each other. Making mistakes and learning from them is how community grows. Help it grow by joining it. A community it not as strong without people willing to bring their honest, broken selves to be a part of it.

I joined a small group in the winter of 2008. A small group is a group that churches run where five to ten people get together and just either participate in a Bible study, play games, or even just sit around and tell stories about their week. At the small group were some of my favorite times of the week. Because it was a safe environment, and once I got used to every one, we would all let loose and laugh so hard it became therapeutic. Not only that, you learn so much when you hear other people talk.

# DEEP INTO THE PSYCHOSIS

Drugs and alcohol are two things that are going to set all your symptoms off, and, depending on the amount you do, they will set you off into a deep or deeper psychosis. I remember being lost and confused deeper than I ever had been once. I had *just* gotten off the drugs and called the Canadian Mental Health Association, and they sent over two workers for me to talk to. As they sat down with me, every second felt like an hour. I would look up to one lady and not say words for a while while I just stared at her. Not knowing I was doing this, I thought I was perfectly fine. Then I would begin to talk and share with them the story of my life that had happened thus far. Nothing excited me, but I was still me deep inside. I felt that what other people were seeing was something different than the real me. I had still had a lot of the same thoughts as to what I did when I did not have bipolar disorder. It drove me nuts that I was all slowed down. I knew I could think faster and be better, but I was so held back. I was never able to say exactly what I wanted to say, and people always seemed to mistake what I really would mean with something else. I could never correct them because either they would move on to the next subject or I wouldn't have any energy to correct them. I hated it. I was a voice trying to be heard, but nothing was coming out. It drove me nuts.

Marya Hornbacher took herself to whole new limits after she drank a lot of alcohol. She would easily drink four bottles of wine at one point. She herself admitted she had become an alcoholic. Read from page 120 to at least page 140 in her book, *Bipolar: Madness,* and read how she describes her thoughts after the alcohol finally sent her bipolar disorder symptoms into a whirlwind like almost none other I have heard before. This should be enough to scare you to not want to drink anymore. But you have to make a firm decision yourself. Have guts. Be strong. You know where to go to for support. It's out there if you need help—support groups, churches. If one church messes around with you, go to another one until you finally find a compassionate one. Leave the church that doesn't accept you, and just forgive them for being humans and making mistakes, and find that church for you. There will be one; I guarantee it. When a soul begins to search, a soul will find. There are hotlines, friends, and families you can call. Hopefully, there will be friends and family for you closeby to talk to. Go to parks and walking trails. Use them to exercise. Read. Don't have money for books? Go to the library to get a book. If you're reading this book, you are one step in the right direction. Keep on reading. Use any resource you have to keep you from things that will pull you down.

## LOSING CONFIDENCE?

What you might not understand is if you choose to lie in bed, even if you are depressed, you're not only wasting time but you're losing your confidence. By losing confidence, it will be harder to get out of bed. I'll admit that today, something was going on with me and has been for the past few days, ever since the beach volleyball tournament I went in. I had felt full of energy since then, but yet every time I sit down to read, a million ideas rush through my head and make me want to pass out, and I instantly do. I had this same problem last year at college, periodically throughout the year. So today, I chose to stay in bed a few extra hours. Then, in the afternoon, I took a four-hour nap. This is odd for me because I haven't napped all summer, unless I missed sleep from the night before; then maybe I would nap. During the school year, seldom was there time for a nap, even if I wanted or needed one. But it all clicked today, after watching the show called *Wife Swap.* One of the fathers in the show had lost his confidence to do anything, so he just cleaned the house all day while his wife worked. If that's your thing, that's fine; but this man, deep inside, wanted to make comics. He just had no confidence to go forth and actually show his comics to prospects who would like to buy them. It took the new wife to tell him that he had no confidence because he didn't do anything that would give it to him.

What I'm saying here is if you're unconfident and you're depressed, you still have to try to do something because that is what battling back is. You can battle back and regain your confidence and your self-worth plus anything else lacking. What you don't realize that even forcing yourself to do a good activity will help. A good activity would be something that is creating peace and possibly pleasing others and pleasing to God, if you believe in him or don't. By doing this activity, what it will do will only boost you, even if you can hardly do it or if you can hardly enjoy it at first. It will boost your self-confidence, which will in return boost your productivity, which may help you feel purpose.

If you like to paint, paint. If you like to write, write. If you like to decorate, do that. Do something that will boost your self-esteem. Oftentimes, throughout history, people who have been depressed usually do some of their best work then because they see things a bit differently, but in a good way. And it might have been hard for Van Gogh to make some of those paintings or Abraham Lincoln to read all those books before he came out of depression and became the president.

It's hard for everyone, and this applies to everyone who is just plain out of motivation like the guy in *Wife Swap.* Keep going. Your dreams can be your reality if you fight through the pain.

# GETTING RID OF STRESS

Not being stressed out is crucial to living a good life. If you have bipolar disorder, supposedly stress builds up on you fast and you can't handle much stress at all. That's why it's considered a disability to have bipolar disorder, because many can't work. Depending how far along you are in your recovery, your stress levels will be different. Your mind will be different, and the way you handle stress will be different.

To get rid of stresses, try acting. Whether it's just some improv with some friends or just randomly making a play up in your head, it can be a great release of stress. Try dancing. Laughter is the best way to get rid of stress for me and a lot of others I have spoken to, but laughing can be included with the activities I mentioned above. Laughing should be included in most of your daily activities. Obviously, use wise discretion when laughing. If you are working in an office building, laughing the whole 8 hours may not be the most courteous thing to your employer.

I was in my brother's room one day, helping him make his bed. He's twelve, but it's hard to make his bed because he has a bunk bed. I was feeling pretty tensed at the moment. And we were just talking, and I made this weird movement with my head, and a weird noise come from my mouth with it. I felt it released a lot of stress. I thought, *Wow! I must look kind of funny doing this.* I did it when Dale, my brother, wasn't looking. Then I asked him what it looked like. "Seizure maybe?" I asked him. He said, "No. A seizure is on the ground." In my mind, I thought, *What the heck. Like this?* and then fell on the ground and made my body shake around as fast as I could. I figured, hey, if I ever need to act in a movie one day where my character needs to have a seizure, I will be prepared. It felt great! I could hear Dale laughing in the background, which made it even better because now I was laughing with someone and letting loose all my energy at the same time.

Then he and I got kind of carried away. We made it into a play. The reason we made it into a play is because Dale said, "What if you were actually having one and I was just laughing, and you just died and I thought I was still playing around and went to bed and said good night." I laughed with him at that thought. Then we thought it would be funny to go downstairs and show this play to my mother.

So we came downstairs in character; then I just started having the seizure right in front of my mom on the kitchen floor. We sort of forgot to introduce that this was a play. I finally stopped the seizure, going into dying mode, and that's when I could hear my mom screaming. She told me to never fake that again.

Dale and I both agreed that next time we would introduce the play as a play rather than give ole mom the scare of her life. The good news is she thought it was real, so, Hollywood, if you need an actor to play a seizure, I'm all for it. And I have a good reference too.

Maybe you can relate to me if you're bipolar and it seems there's always drama wherever you go. Maybe you can relate to me if you're human about that fact. If you understand this, let me tell you right now that if you keep working through recovery—taking your meds, being thankful, loving, giving, learning, exercising, breathing, being creative, staying away from drugs and alcohol, living a life of endurance—then all that drama and all that stress you can't handle seems to diminish.

I mean it. I have experienced it firsthand. When my bipolar disorder symptoms started getting really bad, I didn't realize it. I was just self-medicating whatever problems I seemed to be having with marijuana. I seemed to attract trouble too! In that short period of time, I was pulled over by the cops eight times. Five times, I got tickets.

That's not the best example. The best is when my school turned on me, I went from a guy everyone knew and seemed to respect. Now, I look back to right around the time bipolar disorder hit. All my close friends sort of went away from me. People would write, "Taff's a goof," "F*** Taff," and other coarse, random insults all over the school. They even vandalized my car.

I don't know why this part of my story is always the hardest for me to talk about. One another occasion, at the after-grad party, I remember being there, high on marijuana of course—it was that point of my life where I was usually on drugs—I didn't say much the whole time I was there. I looked around. I saw all the boys by the campfire. I sat down with them for awhile. I still didn't say much. The fire was warm. I could feel it right on my face. I walked over to a guy who had never been to parties before. He was considered a loser at school for the most part, and that's how it seemed people felt about him at the time anyways. He was cutting wood. I said to him; "Hey . . . " I can't remember my words or his back to me. Then he just looked away and kept cutting the wood. Did I ever move away from him cutting that wood? I don't know. I don't know what happened. I was so lost, so confused.

Jason, a friend, stood by me. He talked to me, and I exchanged words with him. Then someone started making fun of Jason. I forget if they were making fun of me too. I was scared though. I did not know what was happening. I don't know how seven men came to the conclusion to try to beat me down. I had done nothing. Or was that it? Had I done nothing? Was I supposed to have done something? I had no problem with these guys or anybody. What was happening? Why had they swarmed around me? Why was he yelling at me in front of everyone to leave? Why were they so mad? Why were the people mad at me at school enough to write my name and insults beside my name on all the benches? Why was I alone? Where was my escape? I managed to get away from the guys that night, but the thoughts kept racing. What was happening? What mattered?

Unfortunately, and sometimes fortunately, I'm a guy who doesn't always find the answer immediately. I often learn the hard way. When it's all gone and nothing matters anymore, that is when God came into the center of my life. I had nothing else. He found me. I guess I was available to be found then.

While I still had clothes and food, inside, I was dead, dying on the street. *This is what it feels to walk again?* I questioned as God started to help me walk again. It was as if life was a dark tunnel I had been sliding down and now I was at the bottom and I could see the light. Truth was in this light. It was quite lovely. My flesh hated it. It tried to lie, saying this wasn't good. But being in the light was like having a constant hug because he's always there, and I was beginning to be accepting of that. While I still have bipolar disorder, I now have light and direction. While I still have stress, I have witnessed healing take place in my life.

Now, when I'm around people, I still feel like that drama is lurking, but it's rarely against me and it's usually about who left the milk out—things that we can deal with. I felt a little bit of tension, but a whole lot of hope. I have seen my life heal up. I see that I'm healing, learning, and being renewed daily. I have faith I won't stop being healed because I believe in Jesus.

I believe in his miracles. I believe he can do anything. I believe his Father created us all. It breaks my heart when I hear people who don't believe in him. I was lost, but now I am found. Thank you, Jesus. If you ask me honestly what gets me through my days, my belief in God does. I would be on the street, homeless right now if it wasn't for him. He gave me hope. Everybody needs hope, especially when they're suffering. Suicide rates would decrease, guaranteed, if we had hope. God tells us he will not give us anything we cannot handle (1 Corinthians 10:13). Jesus provides comfort. When you reject the comfort, how can he give it to you? How can the poor, homeless man with broken legs get up unless he allows someone to give him a hand up?

God coming to me was like I was in a coma, and he finally woke me up. How could I have not seen? It's so clear now. It makes so much sense. It's all lined up so perfect, the same as how two plus two equals four. If you have accepted money before, why can't you accept Jesus? It makes money worth accepting.

It's as if you're standing close to a tornado and all the objects flying at you bring you no fear because each object represents a blessing from God and they hit you hard. Clarity may come natural to you, but, to me, it came as a blessing. Maybe you're blessed with natural peace; maybe not. I pray that you don't have to find lessons out the hard way. Maybe you're generous to the poor. That means nothing to God if you don't believe in him.

I'm not asking how you could deny your creator, but I'm sure God is. He knows Satan and realizes this punk is pulling too many lies over your heads. If Jesus couldn't wake you up when he died for you after fulfilling Old Testament prophecies, healing the sick and lame, forgiving the very people who persecuted him, and for living life harming nobody and still being beat down for no reason at all, then how am I supposed to? I am just a human like you. It is the bad experiences in my life that have driven me closer to Jesus. In the book *Pursuit of God* by Tozer, Tozer spends almost a whole chapter just talking about how God has a personality and how we can discover it. Man, do I want to discover it, and I am discovering it, and the colors are much brighter in here, and I'm not talking about being elated either. I'm talking about real life. Billy Graham gave almost the whole world a chance to accept Jesus through his questions. Still, people said no. Are you going to say no like everyone else? Fear or no fear, you must make a decision and not regret it. The opportunity is there. Please join me.

# DEALING WITH YOUR CHILD WHO MAY HAVE HAD BIPOLAR DISORDER FROM THE TIME OF THE WOMB

Ever since I was a baby, something was different about me, my mom and I realized, looking back on my life. After my mom and I read, *Parenting a Bipolar Child* By Gianni L Faded, MD, and Nancy B. Austin, PSYD, we realized I was possibly bipolar the day I was born. My mom says, "One hundred percent, not a doubt in my mind, you were bipolar as a kid." This was huge to me, seeing how I wrote 75 percent of this book, thinking bipolar disorder did not come to me until grade ten or eleven. I never really thought I was bipolar from birth. I thought it came when I was in grade ten or eleven. The reason I thought this was because I was happier during those younger ages. But looking back and having my mom recount stories to me that proved her point made me realize I *may* have been. We came to the definite conclusion that, while I may have been bipolar as a kid, it definitely peaked in grades ten and eleven with my symptoms. Even in the mom's womb, I was always active, kicking and turning constantly.

My mom recounted incidents to me that may have proven her point. We started off by picking out all the symptoms I had as a child, and they were irritability, rudeness, temper tantrums, argumentativeness, being full of rage, having problems falling asleep at night, brightness, being creative and talented, hyperactivity, distractibility, pressured speech, being too fast and loud, impulsiveness, and having trouble functioning at school. Then, for every point, she gave me a story to prove her point.

Some of the following techniques my mom attempted and can be used for you as well while dealing with a child with bipolar disorder. There is a general idea in each story that can be used as a guideline, but the strategy you develop will need to be geared to your own child.

For a child with bipolar disorder, it can be especially difficult experiencing extreme emotions at such a young age when it's hard to comprehend. A child may feel hopeless or scared and become out of control for no reason at all. A simple no from parents can set a bipolar child off, or a very stimulated area will overstimulate a bipolar child and they will become so high in emotions and energized that they won't know how to come down.

Oftentimes, as a young child, from age one to age four, before I really developed a sense of self-control and firm set of morals, knowing what is right or wrong, I would hit people, even adults. My mom observed that I would get so energized, so excited, and all that would start off as fun; then the person I was playing with in the highly stimulated area (such as a party) would start to calm down, and as a young could, I would not know how to calm down. I would be so pumped up I might just whack the person right in the face or some similar action.

The doctors say there is not much comfort you can give a child when he is out of control. My mom found this to be true with me. Nothing seemed to calm me down or comfort me. But sometimes I would get so energetic that she was concerned for someone else's safety or my own safety. In that case, she would (only in a private area; she did not want to humiliate me in a public area) squeeze me with the biggest hug she could possible give me and not let go and let me have my temper tantrum in her arms. Apparently, this would wear me out, and I would finally go limp in her arms.

I'm told I was spanked a lot. My parents would discipline me with everything and not let me get away with anything. The discipline seemed to work, and my mom always told me never to hit anyone, no matter what, and after four or so, when I really started grasping that concept, I never did hit anyone again, until my fight in grade nine.

Oftentimes, as a child from age one to four, I would also freak out and hit or hurt when I felt that people got in my space. Adults would always want hugs and would make me hug them, even when I didn't want one, and what they didn't know was there was probably a good reason I didn't want a hug—probably because I was to pumped up and focused and a hug just wouldn't be good at the moment. One time, at age two or three, my aunt tried to hug me, and, regretfully, I scratched her.

## Bipolar In Adolescents

Like I have pointed out earlier in the book, the onset of Bipolar is from age eighteen to age twenty-or, or from age thirty to age forty. But a lot of people close to me who knew me when I was younger are starting to notice that, yes, maybe I did have it at a younger age. Like I said earlier, for me, who thinks it's quite possible and to my mom, who is almost certain that I had bipolar disorder as a young kid, it is evident to anyone who knew me that the symptoms did not increase to a noticeable and more excruciating amount for me until grade ten or eleven.

Some researchers believe that the onset could come for some people in their adolescence (their early teens). It's usually very hard to notice though, because you must differ between a regular rebellious teen and one who is irritable and moody. While a rebellious teen might argue with his or her parents or any authoritative figure, one who has bipolar disorder, will seem like all they're spitting out of their mouth are arguments to these types of people.

While I have always been slightly argumentative, what I'm trying to describe here—which is more extreme than being a slight arguer—did come out of me to my teachers in high school in, for sure, grade eleven. My friend, told me years later that all I did was argue with teachers. I hardly remember this. I do slightly, but I don't recall them as arguments in my head. But I will admit they probably were. Looking back, the arguments were probably a cry for help. This is good to know if you notice this in teens that are ever in your life.

Now, if I did have bipolar disorder as a kid, that would definitely mean I had it during my adolescence. Let's see. Did I have problem with authority as a child? Well, I certainly didn't directly argue with the teachers because I was thinking I had an authority problem with them, but through my actions, it was apparent that either I was trying to have a lot of fun or quite possibly, somewhere in there, I may have slightly had a problem with authority—at least with my teachers anyways. At times, we, as people, may have a problem we are unaware of, and that was the case for me.

My behavior and emotions were all right in my grade eight year, to begin with. We had a nice teacher. Mr. R, we will call him. Then he had some health problems, so he had to leave and substitutes had to fill in. Que the horror music please because that's what it turned into from here on in, horror.

I did it with a smile the whole time though. I wasn't showing much moodiness, but we sure brought the drama, and it wasn't just me; it was the whole entire class—all of them, some worse then others, but at one point, everyone did something wrong. (I'm almost certain.); even the kid who told on me for having a pocket knife and Chinese fire crackers at school, which, by the way, I forgot the knife in my pocket from the day before out in the woods, and, yes, all my clothes were dirty, so I wore the same pair twice. It wasn't like I was going to stab any body. Seriously, I'm not one to carry knives around normally. But, yes, even you were having fun, person who told on me. When? you ask. Well, I sure didn't see you putting up much of a fight when we turned Mr. W's class into a dance party.

Yes, we moved all the desks aside, someone actually had a disco light, and we put on the beats and were dancing in the middle of class. Poor guy didn't know what to do. He didn't want to go to the principal—he would look bad as a teacher—so he just gave in, and then, finally, he had enough and turned off the music. That was an hour or so into the party. What a math class that was.

Well, that's only one incident, you say, although that's quite intense. Isn't there any chance you might not have had bipolar disorder? Well, my *childhood* stories really tell it all, but I'll go on to tell you more about the grade eight year.

You see, that was only one teacher who was overrun. We went through thirteen different teachers. We could have gotten to twenty, but the last teacher, the thirteenth, had to sign a contract stating he wouldn't leave. The guy was a former bouncer, for crying out loud. The principal and other teachers thought for sure we were going to respect him. Did we? No. I have never seen anybody leave so fast on the last day of school in my life. Usually, kids run pretty fast, but this guy beat the kids out the door.

As funny as it all seems, we were disrespectful, and that's the only part we went wrong with. We may have handled the voicing of our needs a bit inappropriately. I believe we are to respect authority no matter what. And if they aren't just, then we justly rise above the system and put them back where they belong—God willing, of course.

I'm not saying the teachers were never wrong. We put them through madness, so all my mercy goes out to all of them. I'm sorry. I truly am. But I would like to say one thing to a few of you who took it upon yourselves to tell a few of us that we would never make it anywhere in life, that we would never amount to anything in life. While I agree we were out of hand, and I know things slip, but telling a young kid that is the opposite of what you're supposed to do. Honestly, I don't know what would have stopped us. We were ruthless, filling the empty desks with all the crust from our sandwiches; putting eggs with holes in them in there, trying to stink out the classroom; making loud noises every time the teacher turned his or her back, leaving him or her trying to figure out who did it while we took turns all throughout the classroom, making it impossible to nail one person. Man, we did it all. We were never violent and rough. Maybe a few guys once or twice out in the field got a bit rowdy. We were all, dare I say it, good kids—most of us anyways. Some just through even me for a whirl with the stuff they did. But, yes, I did not stop wreaking havoc. No way will I claim I did most of it. That would take too many kids' glory away who are proud of what they had done, but I will say put away the past; look to the present; and, yes, you can do it.

I got good sleep during my adolescence. I biked, I swam, I played computer games quite obsessively—I seemed like a normal kid if you ask me. It would be really hard to tell if I was bipolar, but I must have been if I was as a child. My closest friends will tell you though that the huge changes occurred in my tenth and eleventh-grade years.

## Treatments for Kids and Adolescents

Would treatment have helped if I had it before things got out of hand in grades ten and eleven and so on? When we talk about treatment in kids and adolescents doctors often will talk about things like pacing a child's day and week, not overstimulating the child. My mom already figured this out in me when I was a child and would watch that she didn't *always* bring me to big events. As I grew older in my adolescence, parties, family gatherings, and other stimulating places weren't so bad because I had more self-control and was smarter and wiser. So it really takes good parents to be in tune with their kids as a best source of treatment. The best thing you can do, parents, to help the situation, is make your kid aware of what they may have and educate them on it. Why? Because of this: one thing that every person with illnesses needs is insight. You cannot have insight into your illness until you accept that you have the illness, and then, once you have accepted that, you can become aware of what's happening to you and you begin to have insight. If one knows what's happening to him, he can do what's best for him. Even young kids can become aware of the moods that they're having. Young girls with bipolar disorder often will articulate, "My thoughts are racing." If they knew perhaps why, they may feel better and know how to go on with the next thought instead of feeling lost after the thought, *My thoughts are racing.* They can continue with the possible thought process, *I have bipolar disorder. What is bipolar disorder? Where does it come from? How did I get it? Who else has it? How did they deal with it?* Then they can read this book, depending on their reading level or if they can read at all because, basically, if you can read, you can read this book and realize that there is *hope* for them. Once your child has hope, there is nothing stopping them. Just help harness their energy and be there for them every second you can, in heart, in physical presence, or in prayer. An open parent who tries to understand their child's illness is comforting for the child. It will remove a huge block between you and your child. Never stop praying for your child. Their illness is too big for anyone. The only way is giving it to God. There are many other things you can do, but give it to God first and let other things follow. I have heard of too many stories of kids rejecting their parents, usually because they don't find out they have bipolar disorder until they hit rock bottom, or they reject their parents even if they do know because their illness is too difficult for them and they think their parents are making it worse.

The story of the prodigal son in the Bible reminds me of a great story for you, if you are a parent and especially if your child has left you and stopped talking to you because of his or her illness. You should be like the parent of the prodigal son, a story I'm going to share with you because it will be the biggest blessing to your kid and fulfill you as a parent.

And for parents whose kids haven't left them but it still seems difficult because they are being violent and hurting others, and even their siblings, or they're just sleeping all the time and you're sad for them, give them something that will comfort them, a good story and good book, love, grace, and blessings. Bipolar is evil, and if you look at it that way, just fight evil with what it hates: love. I understand a lot of bipolar people can be very creative, but, to me, that has got to be God's gift for us having to go through what we do. But the negative symptoms can be deleted if you believe.

## The Prodigal Son (Luke 11–32)

> Jesus continued: "There was a man who had two sons. The younger one said to his father, 'Father, give me my share of the estate.' So he divided his property between them.
>
> "Not long after that, the younger son got together all he had, set off for a distant country and there squandered his wealth in wild living. After he had spent everything, there was a severe famine in that whole country, and he began to be

in need. So he went and hired himself out to a citizen of that country, who sent him to his fields to feed pigs. He longed to fill his stomach with the pods that the pigs were eating, but no one gave him anything.

"When he came to his senses, he said, 'How many of my father's hired men have food to spare, and here I am starving to death! I will set out and go back to my father and say to him: "Father, I have sinned against heaven and against you. I am no longer worthy to be called your son; make me like one of your hired men."' So he got up and went to his father.

"But while he was still a long way off, his father saw him and was filled with compassion for him; he ran to his son, threw his arms around him and kissed him.

"The son said to him, 'Father, I have sinned against heaven and against you. I am no longer worthy to be called your son.'

"But the father said to his servants, 'Quick! Bring the best robe and put it on him. Put a ring on his finger and sandals on his feet. Bring the fattened calf and kill it. Let's have a feast and celebrate. For this son of mine was dead and is alive again; he was lost and is found.' So they began to celebrate.

"Meanwhile, the older son was in the field. When he came near the house, he heard music and dancing. So he called one of the servants and asked him what was going on. 'Your brother has come,' he replied, 'and your father has killed the fattened calf because he has him back safe and sound.'

"The older brother became angry and refused to go in. So his father went out and pleaded with him. But he answered his father, 'Look! All these years I've been slaving for you and never disobeyed your orders. Yet you never gave me even a young goat so I could celebrate with my friends. But when this son of yours who has squandered your property with prostitutes comes home, you kill the fattened calf for him!'

"'My son,' the father said, 'you are always with me, and everything I have is yours. But we had to celebrate and be glad, because this brother of yours was dead and is alive again; he was lost and is found.'"

# TWO SUFFERERS LIVING TOGETHER

My mom and I living together was always difficult. It still can be. When I come back from school in the summer and visit my family, it's hard with my mom. I take most the responsibility on my own shoulders. I figured if I could just learn to cope in tough situations better I would make it through. You see, my mom has degenerate disc disease, fibromyalgia and some kind of mood disorder. And with her mother just dying, she is in an all-time low of her life. She describes it as a living hell.

I'm going to tell you right now, straight up, that it is harder to be compassionate to a family member in pain than a stranger. Why? Not sure. Maybe because you see the person every day complaining about the same thing. Nothing you do is right for the person. And I say it's harder for me because, whatever the cause, I'm sighing like crazy, overwhelmed with everything that's going down in my own life. Then my mom starts to sigh, and I hear her sigh and I get more stressed and my sighs just become normal breathing of hopelessness and despair, and then she sees the absolute terror pain in my eyes and gets even worse her self; then we just start to get mad at each other and irritated with each other. It's so messed up.

I know I love my mom and she deserves every ounce of love I give her and more. It's just that the headache and fight is so hard, almost unlivable. "What do you have me up against, God?" I yell. It's weird. You think I would just get sick of her and leave, but I keep coming back to her and I keep longing to talk to her because once you get through the pain and possibly get your space and think about what has just happened, you realize that she may have inspired you the most. Love is hard because love lasts, and that means you have to last with it, and that means being there for every second of the drive. No matter how much you want to open the front door and hurl yourself out, you can't. You must stay buckled up and endure the race. Keep your mama safe and protect her. She's a fountain of knowledge and wisdom for you to drink of, and I won't go too far without thanking my dad. He's a superhero! Remember one thing as you go through it all: it's all worth it in the end. I love my mom. And every day, God heals us both and is bringing us to complete redemption within our broken souls.

## ENDURE

So you have listened to everything I have said in this book and more and you still lie in bed with an empty feeling in your chest that leaves you feeling lonely and lost. You're still confused. Pain won't leave you alone. You're begging for it to go away, but it won't go away. You keep enduring. You pursue patience, your best friends, with hope, but you're breaking down. You can't take the pain any more. *What more do I have to do?* you think. *I put away the alcohol, I put away the drugs, I put away all the premarital sex*... Your thoughts race. *The meds I'm taking, why aren't they working?* You question. Everything in you feels filled up with sorrow, but crying isn't even good enough. Nothing is going your way. You're tired, and you want rest. You keep walking. You keep doing the right thing. Thank you. You're officially my hero.

It takes a hero to do what you're doing, to say no to everything that might make you feel better for a second; instead, you trade it in for dignity, healthy pride, and respect. You use your strength to lift others up while you go ahead and suffer. You will succeed, but even the thought of success doesn't lift you up. For men and women like you, there is only one thing I can give you that might help you, and that is the promise that there is a place full of no pain, where you can live. We can't imagine or grasp how good it will be because we have never experienced anything like it. If you endure and do the work you're supposed to do, the prize is even bigger, but if you only "confess with your mouth Jesus is lord and believe in your heart that God raised him from the dead you will be saved," (Romans 10:9). If you feel like there is nothing in this world for you, this is most definitely for you. It's for all, but if you can relate to this, you're probably feeling me in this instance when I say that God can satisfy. If you looked around and said, "Nah. This just isn't it. This just can't be it, man—dirty proposals being pursued through the underground child sex trade, open wounds having salt poured on them, empty hollowness and sorrow-filled hearts when I wake and when I sleep. Nah. This just can't be it. Let's forget it, but, man, I got to keep marching on." I cry, and my tears pour out to you right now. I can only stop myself from not crying constantly because I know that there's a place we can go together and be happy, and that's it! I don't care what you say. I'm going there, and I'm not looking back. You're either coming with me or you're not. It's your choice, and I can't change that. If I could, I'd slap you up right and make you come with me, because if this isn't hell, then I really Want Gods vengeance to go out on Satan.

You can't tell satan to burn in hell because he is hell. He likes it there. He is pain, and he hates us because God loves us. Like a civilian in a war zone running to a safe zone, let's do what we got to do. Don't look back. Put away the pride, please. I know you can. We need hope and mercy. Believe me, believe yourself because of what you already know. If you have lived more than one minute and definitely more then one day, you know there's something not right here on earth. As soon as the baby comes out, he starts to cry. He doesn't even like it here. He just learns to live with it and then tries to make the best of it like we all do. Let's go to a better place together. Some call it heaven; some call it home.

## SHED A TEAR

It takes a true soldier to cry. Crying does not make you weak. It should never be looked at like that or laughed at because for a man or woman to cry means he or she is doing one thing right; he or she is releasing his or her strife, anger, and all his or her pain the natural way. It is much better to be angry and use self-control to control the anger to the point it brings you to tears than to act out on your anger. As life hands out its shares of burdens, sometimes releasing our stress through the normal opening of tear ducts is what we have to do; it's what it takes to save a man's life.

# THEY ALL HATE YOU!

A common thought I hear not only from Bipolar Individuals but from anyone who has done acts they may be shamed about is that people who are not doing those acts—and possibly rich, preppie families may get blamed for this the most—is that people such as I described hate people like me (*Madness, a Bipolar Life,* 2008 Marya Hornbacher). People who have stolen and still do steal; or have done drugs or still do drugs; or prostitute or still do give sex for money; or people who lie, cheat, and hurt all carry a heaven burden that does not need to be carried once they have stopped. So if you're bipolar and you have done things in your past that you have hated and despised in yourself and you are stuck in the ugly triple trap of guilt and fear and self-hatred, also more specifically occupied by fear that others hate you because of things you have done, you need to know its not what people think but what God thinks. It may be true others may hate people like you, they may despise you, ridicule you and want to take you out like the Wednesday morning trash, you may have to accept this. They may not even have to know who you are or the exact individual you are, and what you do for fun; they just turn their heads the other way when you pass. It's important to know that it's only what God thinks of you. We are all to love each other as Christ has loved us.

I don't want to even bring up the obvious fact that we have all stolen and done things that we think people hate us for, which would make whoever hate us hypocrites, the biggest one being Satan. I do not really need to bring that up because that's not good enough, that will not take your shame away, that will not make you feel loved. I cannot even fully make you happy by telling you that I still love you despite what you have done or still do. Because I am only human and my heart cannot consume enough love to fill you, the only thing I can do—and this is the only thing I can do because it's the only thing that matters, and this thing will take away your hatred hopefully for yourself and hopefully give you perspective on the people who hate you but act as if they are perfect—is tell you that they need help from you. That is that Jesus Christ, the son of God, came to earth, and who did he choose to associate himself with? The poor, prostitutes, thieves, tax collectors, demon-possessed the blind, sinners (Matthew 9:32). Who did he eat with? Tax collectors and sinners (Matthew 9:10). Who did he protect in the hardest of times? He protected widows and prostitutes. Who did he elect to teach his powerful message once he died? A murderer, a killer of Christians, Paul the apostle himself. We are all guilty of not being perfect. We all need Jesus. No one is worse or better than the other. We are all God's children.

Why would Jesus come here just to do that for all of you? Because "those who are well don't need a doctor, but the sick do," (Matthew 9:12). Jesus went on to say, "Go and learn what this means: I desire mercy and not sacrifice. For I didn't come to call the righteous but sinners," (Matthew 9:13). He also said, "Blessed are those who mourn; they will be comforted," (Matthew 5:4). No matter who you are, we are instructed in the Bible not to judge, and it's important to know that and know that the only one who can judge is the one who is perfect, and that is Jesus. But he forgives us if we ask him, and he is humble and will accept whoever you are because he loves you and just wants you to accept him. Accepting him is the best thing you can do for yourself in life. Nothing can replace the cross Jesus died on; nothing can bring us closer to Jesus but himself. Call on his name!

## THE DRIVE TO SUCCEED

If you want to make it and survive with bipolar disorder, the drive to succeed and do the best with your life is a must. I find if you're bipolar once you take over the huge duty of changing your ways, mind, and attitude and choose to want to succeed; then you can and will. Your energy, sorrow, or creativity will work with you in this area you are trying to excel at. You too can do it, and not just if you're bipolar. Everyone can spread the news by telling the world that they can do it! They can do all things through Christ, who strengthens them," (Philippians 4:13).

# TO WRAP THINGS UP

To wrap things up here, I care for each and every one of you. I don't know how to help you more than to tell you how I did it. I am still doing it, and I'll also note that I'm constantly looking for new ideas to improve. I will continue to find, hopefully until I die, new ways. All the families out in the world, my heart goes out to you. If you work together, unity can be achieved. To the world, if we all work together, unity is possible. "Everything is possible through Christ" (Philippians 4:13). Bumps and cracks in the road are going to be there, but it's the tires you choose to get across them that are going to make the difference. Christ is there for you whenever you need him. I lean on him for everything I do, and he has yet to let me fall. Open your heart and let Jesus touch it. Pray for everybody. If we all start doing that, a difference will be made. Pray for me. As you read this, I need your prayers.

Two men faced off in an arm wrestling match. They were both equally strengthened. But one wrestler had been taking care of his calcium supply while the other hadn't, resulting in the arm wrestler with not enough calcium having his bone break right in half. In the big scheme of things, God is the one who won. He has a great calcium supply; it is called everlasting life. He will snap Satan in two. Don't go to Satan's evil side full of trickery and hate.

Love will heal! Remember this, and go forth with it. I don't want to stop writing to you guys, but know I will always be there for whatever support I can give and is needed at the time. While I now stop writing to you temporarily, my heart and prayers are with you.

My last comment is that you can do all things through Christ, who strengthens you," (Philippians 4:13).

# BIBLIOGRAPHY

Clifford Whittingham Beers. *A Mind That Found Itself, an Autobiography.* March 1908.

"Oversensitivity," 2006–2009. <http://www.2knowmyself.com/emtional_sensitivity>

"National Institutes of Health." U.S. Department of Health and Human Services. February 04, 2009. <http://nimh.nih.gov/health/publications/the-numbers-count-mental-disorders-in-america/index.shtml>

Gannon Murphy. *Voices of Reasons.* Pensylvania, Camp Hill, 1995.

Gianni C, Faded. *Parenting a Bipolar Child.* Oakland, CA: New Harbinger, 2006.

Marya Hornbacher. *Madness: A Bipolar Life.* Boston, Mass: Houghton Mifflin Co., 2008.

Patty Duke, Gloria Honchman. *Brilliant Madness: Living with Manic Depressive Illness.* New York: Bantam Books, 1992.

Understanding Bipolar Disorder Sedo. <http://www.understandingbipolardisorder.com/article.cfm/id/72363>

"HealthyPlace: America's Mental Health Channel." 2000–2009. <http://www.healthyplace.com/>

"Norepinephrine." Wikimedia Foundation Inc. 26 June 2009 <http://en.wikipedia.org/wiki/Norepinephrine>

"Lithium pharmacology." Wikimedia Foundation Inc. 7 July 2009. <http://en.wikipedia.org/wiki/Lithium_pharmacology>

"Lithium Carbonate." Wikimedia Foundation Inc. 18 June 2009. <http://en.wikipedia.org/wiki/Lithium_carbonate>

"Trimipramine." Internet Mental Health. Philip W. Long, M.D. 1995–2008. <http://www.mentalhealth.com/drug/p30-r02.html>

# NOTES

1 Understanding Bipolar Disorder. <http://www.understanding-bipolardisorder.com/article.cfm/id/72363>

2 Patty Duke and Gloria Honchman "Brilliant Madness: Living with Manic Depressive Illness," Bantam Books, Jacket design 1992 One plus studio.

3 Patty Duke and Gloria Honchman "Brilliant Madness: Living with Manic Depressive Illness," Bantam Books, Jacket design 1992 One plus studio.

4 Patty Duke and Gloria Honchman "Brilliant Madness: Living with Manic Depressive Illness," Bantam Books, Jacket design 1992 One plus studio.

5 Patty Duke and Gloria Honchman "Brilliant Madness: Living with Manic Depressive Illness," Bantam Books, Jacket design 1992 One plus studio.

6 Patty Duke and Gloria Honchman "Brilliant Madness: Living with Manic Depressive Illness," Bantam Books, Jacket design 1992 One plus studio.

7 Patty Duke and Gloria Honchman "Brilliant Madness: Living with Manic Depressive Illness," Bantam Books, Jacket design 1992 One plus studio.

8 Patty Duke and Gloria Honchman "Brilliant Madness: Living with Manic Depressive Illness," Bantam Books, Jacket design 1992 One plus studio.

9 Patty Duke and Gloria Honchman "Brilliant Madness: Living with Manic Depressive Illness," Bantam Books, Jacket design 1992 One plus studio.

10 Patty Duke and Gloria Honchman "Brilliant Madness: Living with Manic Depressive Illness," Bantam Books, Jacket design 1992 One plus studio.

11 Patty Duke and Gloria Honchman "Brilliant Madness: Living with Manic Depressive Illness," Bantam Books, Jacket design 1992 One plus studio.

12 Patty Duke and Gloria Honchman "Brilliant Madness: Living with Manic Depressive Illness," Bantam Books, Jacket design 1992 One plus studio.

13 Patty Duke and Gloria Honchman "Brilliant Madness: Living with Manic Depressive Illness," Bantam Books, Jacket design 1992 One plus studio.

14 Clifford Whittingham Beers. *A Mind That Found Itself, an Autobiography.* March 1908.

15 Gannon Murphy. "Voices of Reasons." Pensylvania, Camp Hill, 1995.

16 "Norepinephrine." Wikimedia Foundation Inc. 26 June 2009. <http://en.wikipedia.org/wiki/Norepinephrine>

17 Clifford Whittingham Beers. *A Mind That Found Itself, an Autobiography.* March 1908.

CPSIA information can be obtained
at www.ICGtesting.com
Printed in the USA
LVOW04s0043051115
461188LV00009BA/108/P